About the Safety Institute USA

What We Do:

The Safety Institute USA, Inc., has been providing instructional courses in First Aid, CPR, AED, Blood-borne Pathogens, Emergency Triage and Assessment and safety related courses for over 35 years with certifications meeting job-related requirements. OSHA and other regulatory agencies require training to help prevent accidents through knowledge and hands-on training.

Our courses are made affordable and have easy access through a wide range of businesses, individual instructors and markets, including:

- Oil Field businesses
- Office Store Front Businesses
- Commercial and Industrial industries
- Transportation Companies
- Early Child and day care centers
- Educational Institutions and Universities
- State and Federal Government agencies
- Hospitals, Public and Private
- Dental groups
- Chiropractic Clinics
- Recreation and Athletic Sport groups
- Outdoor and Hunting Groups and organizations
- Public companies
- OEM and other Public Safety municipalities
- Public and Private school systems
- Public and private safety organizations

Why We Make the Difference:

Helping the public to know how to save-a-life shouldn't be scary.

- Over 40 years of teaching and providing training to hundreds of thousands of clients from all backgrounds.
- Always offering the lowest possible price to keep companies in business.
- By allowing more flexibility in courses to meet the needs of the individuals to meet job and time allotments.
- Being able to offer 24/7 support and direct feedback.
- By making the commitment to make sure each student-client knows that making the difference means being the difference.

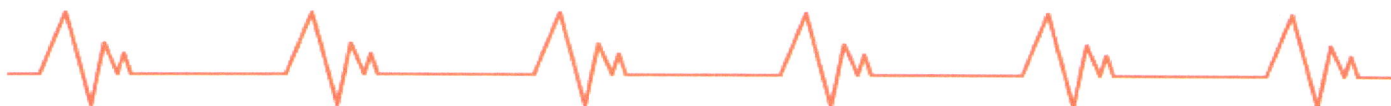

ACKNOWLEDGEMENTS

This manual is dedicated to the many thousands of clients and staff who over the years have made the commitment to change the lives around them by ensuring everyone they touch learns how to save-a-life.

Each course presented is the most current and recognized national and international standards. We recommend all participants; readers and instructors stay informed and updated on changes bi-annually. Our courses are reviewed by professionals in each of these related fields, higher learning, emergency response, occupational health, sports trainers, disaster response, public health and safety, military and emergency response teams.

The Safety Institute USA partners include:

Blas Ramírez
Denise Perry
Larry Allison
Mathew Saavedra
Patty Valle

Debbie Henshaw
Sara Adamo
Robert Coffee
Gordon Hazlett
Tiffany Uresti

Nestor Narveez
Dominick Adamo
Andrea Uresti
Maryann Gonzales
Anthony Cryor

Technical guidance and support

Gilbert R. "Ray" Field
President
Safety Institute USA

Dan Sloan
Developmental Editor

Chris Whitehead, EMT-B
Creative Director

Art, Graphics, Moulage

Susan Calhoun
Moulage

Dan Sloan
Photography

Samantha Jordan
Creative Director

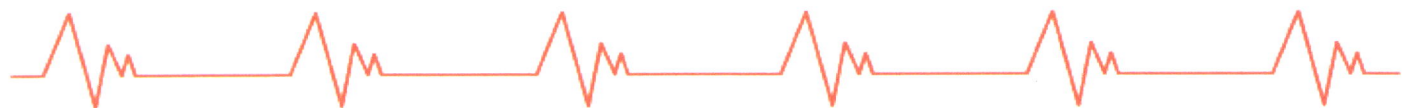

Safety Institute USA

Professional Responders and Health Care

Basic First Aid and Response

CPR – AED Cardiac Emergencies

BBP-Disease-Transmittal Prevention

Oxygen Administration

TODAY

TOMMORROW

EVERYDAY®

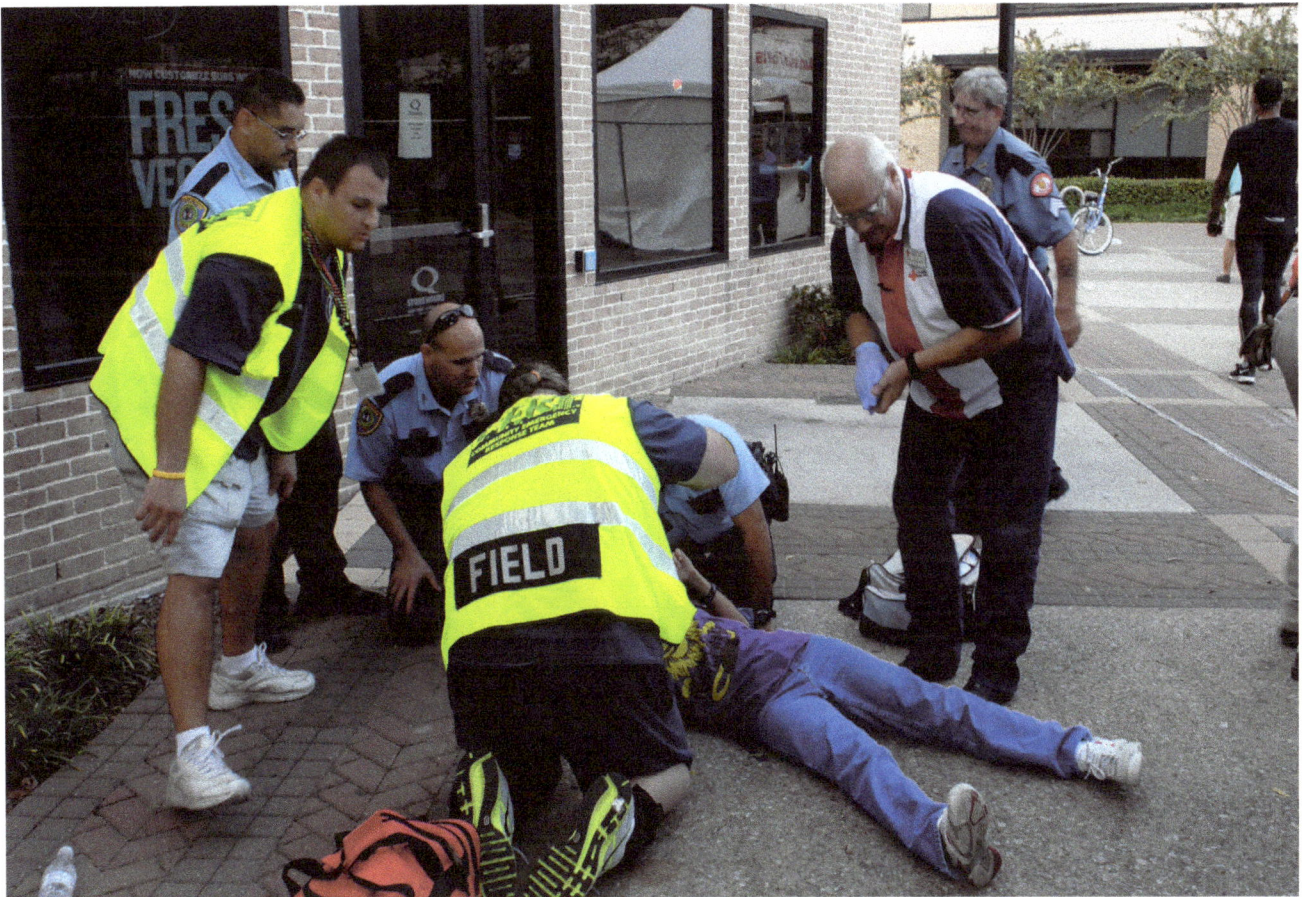

Title: Safety Institute USA Professional Responders and Health Care Basic First Aid Manual by G. R. "Ray" Field

ISBN -13: 9780933316508
Copyright © 2015 by Rolling Olive Press, an imprint of Xenophon Press LLC

7518 Bayside Road, Franktown, Virginia 23354-2106, U.S.A.

XenophonPress@gmail.com

At the time of publication all standards, procedures in this manual reflect the universal standard knowledge and acceptance of emergency practices in the United States and U. S. Territories when published. It is recommended that all participants, readers stay current with up to date changes.

©Safety Institute USA®

Safety Institute USA, Inc.
P. O. Box 692
Franklin, Texas 77856-0692

Email. classes@safetyinstituteusa.org
www.safetyinstituteusa.org
Cover: "First Aid – Patient Down" Photo by Dan Sloan © Copyright 1975-2014 Safety Institute USA.

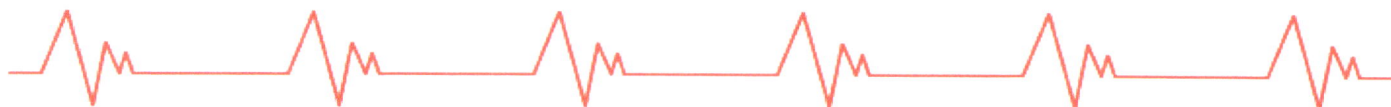

Safety Institute USA
HEALTH AND SAFETY

Professional Responders and Health Care
Basic First Aid and Response
CPR – AED Cardiac Emergencies
BBP-Disease-Transmittal Prevention
Oxygen Administration
CV003-G©2015

Table of Contents

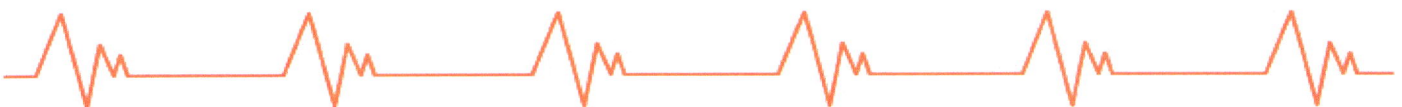

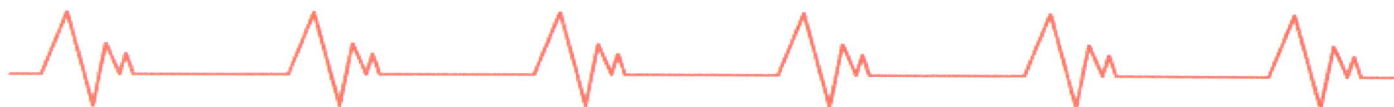

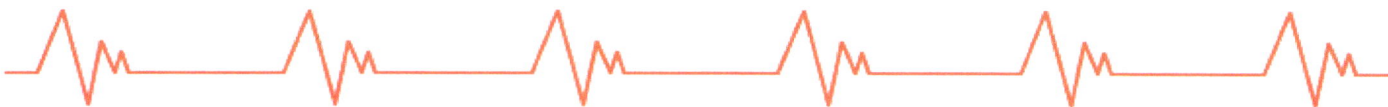

INTENTIONALLY LEFT BLANK

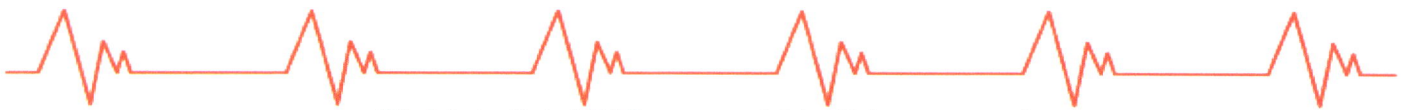

Basic First Aid and Response©

Oxygen Administration

V017-b

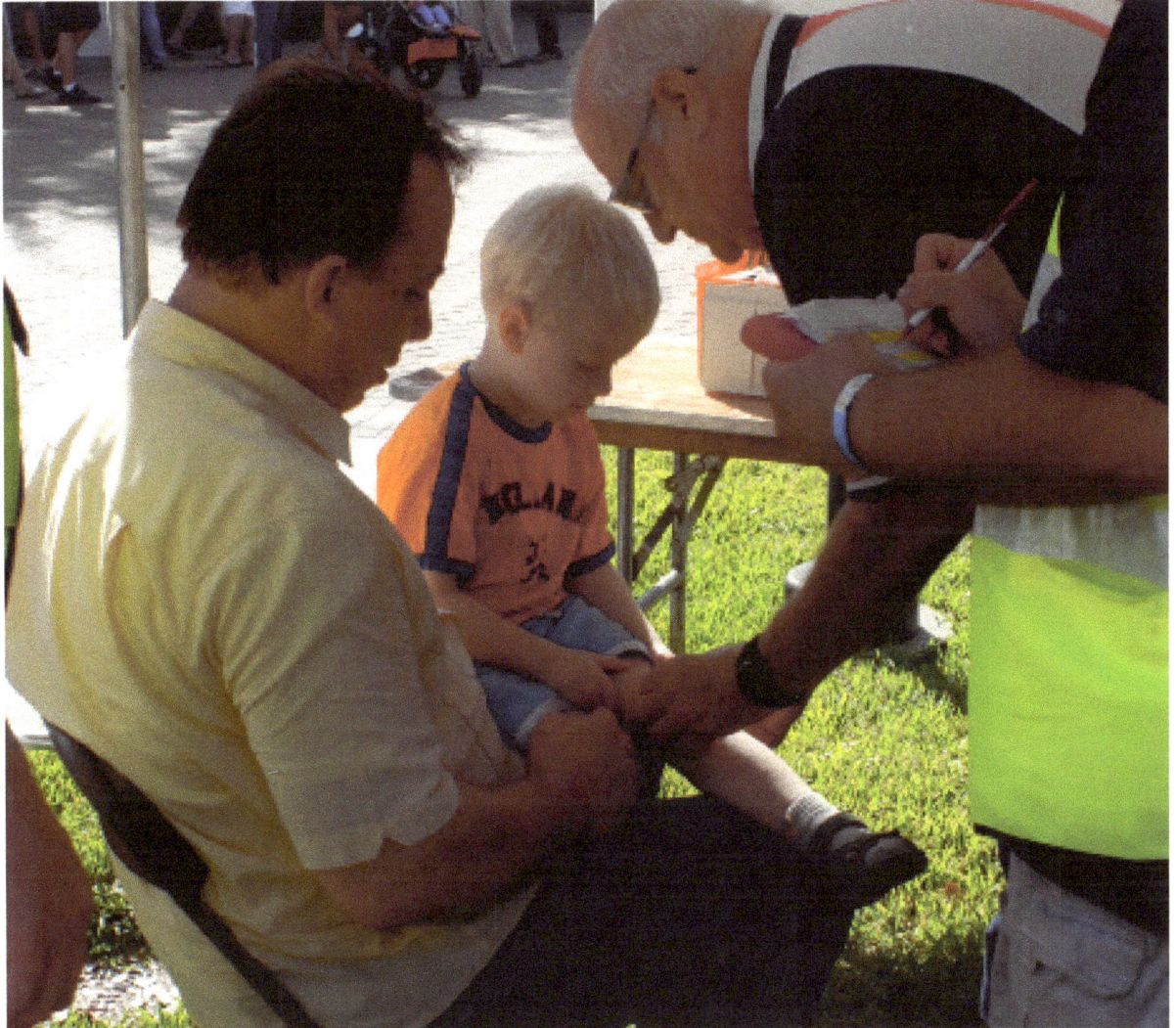

"FIRST AID - SKINNED KNEE"
PHOTOGRAPHER: DAN SLOAN

INTENTIONALLY LEFT BLANK

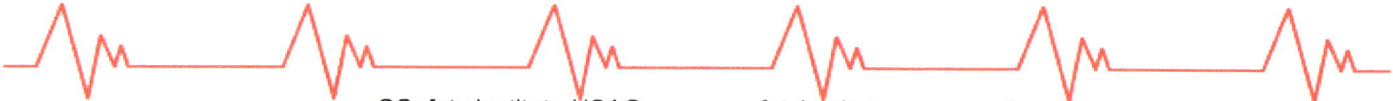

INTRODUCTION

In the workplace, it is often the job of a Certified First Aid Provider to assist in stabilizing an injured or ill person until professional medical help arrives. Certified First Aid Providers are persons who are certified and trained to certain levels in first aid and CPR (Cardiopulmonary Resuscitation). 29 CFR 1910.151(b) states, "In the absence of an infirmary, clinic or hospital in near proximity of the workplace which is used for the treatment of all injured employees, a person or persons shall be adequately trained to render first aid. Adequate first aid supplies shall be readily available."

Good Samaritan Law

Most states have enacted Good Samaritan laws to "encourage" people to help others in emergency situations. These laws give legal protection to people who provide emergency care to ill or injured persons. They require that the "Good Samaritan" use common sense and a reasonable level of skill not to exceed the scope of the individual's training in emergency situations.

If you're interested in learning more about the Good Samaritan laws in your state, contact a local legal professional or check your local library.

Understanding the Principle of First Aid

First Aid by definition means to give care to a person who has a life threatening injury or wound. Understanding that "psychological first-aid" is just as important in healing the victim as treatment.

Lessons learned by the mere value of training and receiving immediate first aid help in lifesaving.

Several factors determine the assistance given when a first aid responder arrives. You may encounter a large number of victims needing assistance, the ever changing environment, the need for proper supplies to assist and ability to have others help.

GLOVES & GLOVE REMOVAL

Personal Protective Equipment is key to minimizing cross contamination. "Latex or Surgical gloves" are important to this process.

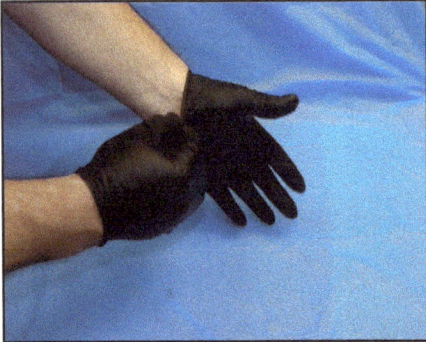

When removing gloves, first pull on the wrist area of the glove so it extends outward.

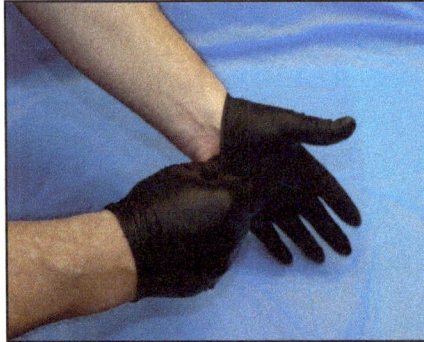

Hook your "thumb" inside the glove. Then pinch glove with index finger to thumb.

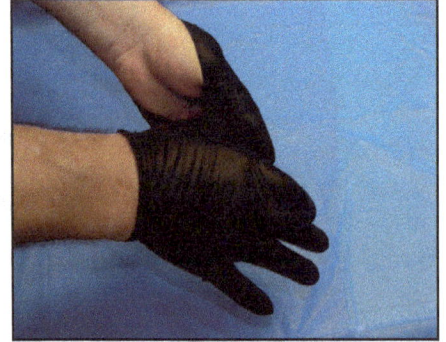

Push thumb downward "rolling" glove down the hand.

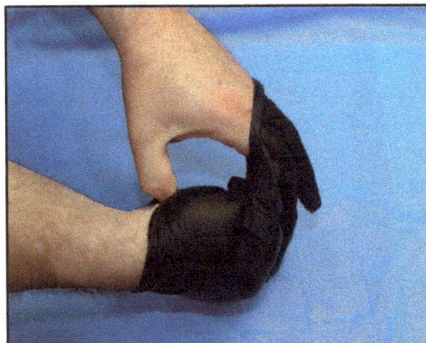

Once glove is rolled off of hand, use "bare thumb" to hook inside other glove.

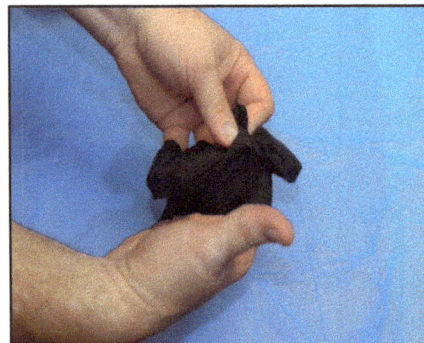

Turn each glove "into themselves" to roll gloves in a ball.

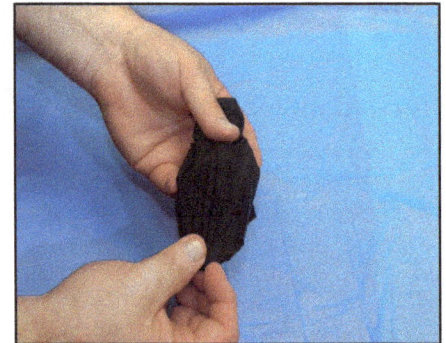

Gloves are turn outside in hiding contaminates from cross contamination.

Proper Disposal of all contaminated materials in "contaminate proof bag" to prevent cross transmission of hazards.

Proper Personal Protective Equipment, Eye-wear, Gloves, Boots, Cover-alls and just a few items to help secure the "hot-zone".

WOUNDS

2 types of wounds typically seen are either Open or Closed.
    "Open Wounds" are breaks in the skin, tears or cuts, lacerations.
    "Closed Wounds" are areas just below the skin where the body has trauma.
Several categories of Open Wounds include:
        Abrasions, Punctures, Avulsions, Incisions, Lacerations
Open Wounds can be caused by hundreds of issues. Primarily these can be found by accidents of car wrecks, bike wrecks, falls, working in the yard.

Abrasions: This is noticed when the skin has been "slightly scared by scraping the body part".
Incisions: The limb or body part has been cut. Handsaws, weed eaters, glass cut, cut by metal.

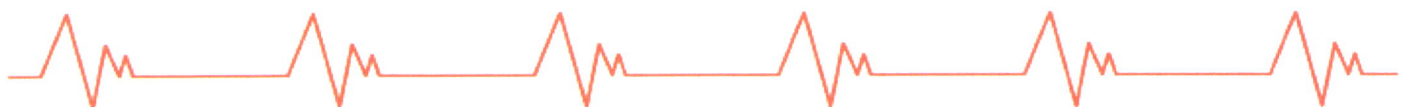

Avulsions: When the part of the body receives a tear in the skin tissue. Cut by knife, ear ring pulled out, dog bite.

Punctures: Whether stepping on a nail, tack or piece of glass. The body receives an object that penetrates the out tissues.

Lacerations: The body has a tear, separation of skin.

ACTION: FIRST AID

In all cases stop the bleeding, fast. Use the cleanest material available.

Put gloves on your hands before contacting the victim. If gloves aren't available then proceed.

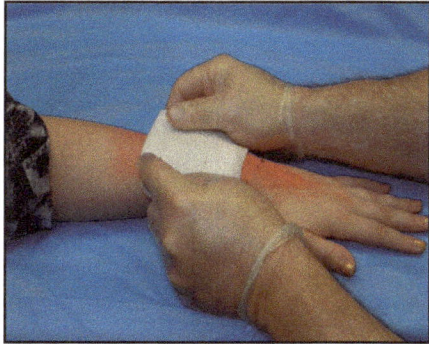

FIRST AID FOR OPEN WOUND

1st. Place first aid dressing material over the top of the wound area.

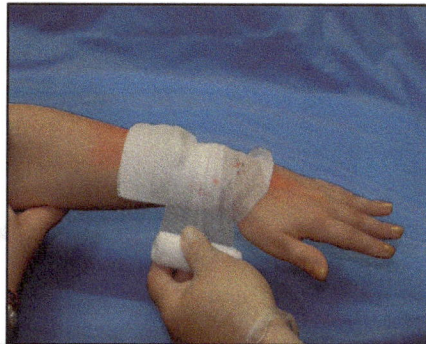

2nd. Tie off material over wound and cover area.

Start by making a "x" with bandage to use tail to cross to secure bandage.

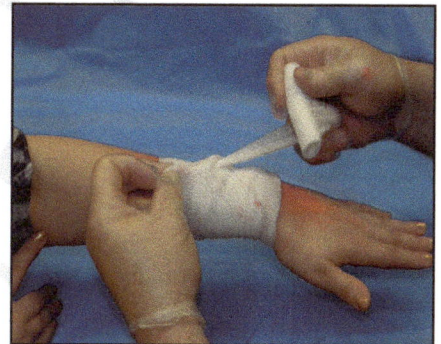

End by tying knot over the top of the "cut" to apply light pressure direct.

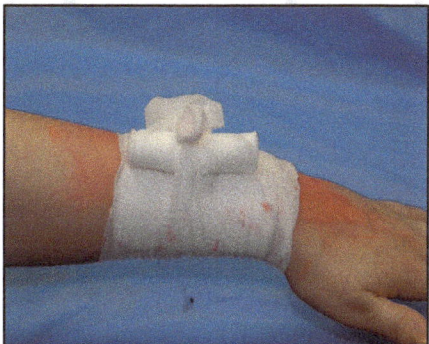

Finish by "tucking-in" the remaining gauze over the cut, under the knot so that if bleeding restarts, you have material to continue.

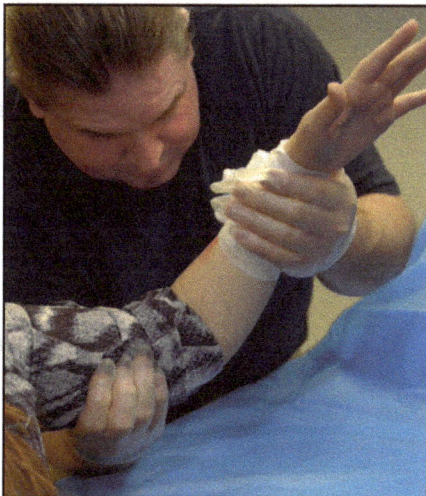

3rd. Elevate the area above the main artery closest to the wound.

Hold wound area up to position.

4th Apply 4 fingers flat against brachial artery, softly until enough pressure has decreased the blood.

5th. Treat for shock

FIRST AID for shock: Keep victim lying still but comfortable. Cover them with a blanket to maintain body temperature. **Call EMS/9-1-1**

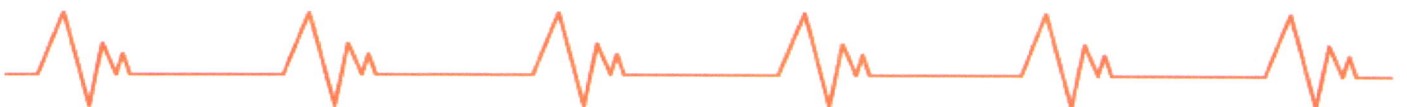

ALLERGIC REACTION

A severe allergic reaction (anaphylaxis) can develop into a life threatening respiratory distress. It comes on within seconds or minutes when an individual is exposed to a specific allergy reaction. Most allergy causing situations can cause this reaction including pollen, bee sting, some foods and drugs, insect venom. Some cases of anaphylactic reaction are of unknown origin.

Some patients break out in hives, watery eyes, swollen lips or face. The muscles around the throat may swell causing swallowing or breathing. Dizziness, mental confusion, cramping, nausea, vomiting may occur with a severe allergic reaction.

Most patients who have had anaphylactic reactions usually carry medications for antidote. Epinephrine is the most widely used drug for severe reactions. This only a temporary fix and medical help is advised immediately.

If you observe someone having and an allergic reaction:

ACTION: FIRST AID

1. Get medical help immediately.

2. Ask patient if they have antidote or special medicine to take, inhale, swallow or inject to counter the effects.

3. If patient becomes unconscious begin rescue steps of CPR.

4. If medicine is not available ask for any histamine to induce while conscious.

Anaphylaxis and Epinephrine Auto-Injector

Recognizing the signs of respiratory emergencies is critical. Key first indicator is called, "Anaphylaxis Shock".

What are Symptoms of Anaphylaxis?

Anaphylaxis may begin with minor itching to severe itching of the face, eyes, swollen lips and upper body. In just minutes it can spread to more serious symptoms including hard to swallow, difficult to breath, hive, cramps, abdominal pains and vomiting.

If you have or see someone with symptoms of anaphylaxis get emergency medical help immediately.

What are common signs of Anaphylaxis?

Generally FOOD is the most common cause of anaphylaxis. Others like shellfish, shrimp-lobster, dairy products, nuts, bee or wasp stings cause anaphylaxis.

Medications can cause anaphylaxis.

Outdoor pollens or inhaled allergens rarely cause anaphylaxis.

Known treatments for Anaphylaxis?

Epinephrine by Injection is the fastest most effective treatment for allergic reactions. Epinephrine may produce symptoms and signs that include an increase in heart rate, the sensation of a more forceful heartbeat, palpitations, sweating, nausea and vomiting, difficulty breathing, pallor, dizziness, weakness or shakiness, headache, apprehension, nervousness or anxiety. These symptoms and signs usually subside rapidly, especially with rest, quiet and recumbence.

In case of accidental injection, the patient should be advised to immediately go to the emergency room for treat ment. Since the epinephrine in the EpiPen Auto-injector is a strong vasoconstrictor when injected into the digits, hands or feet, treatment should be directed at vasodilatation if there is such an inadvertent administration to these areas.

If you are near someone who is going into anaphylactic shock, call for professional medical help immediately. CPR and other lifesaving measures may be required.

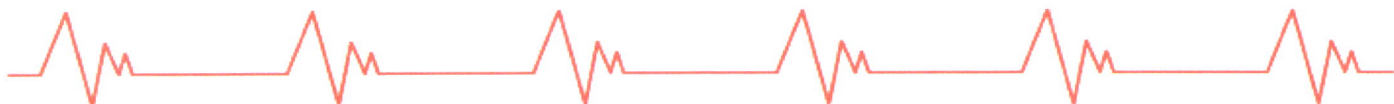

If Your Victim;

Has an "Epi-pen" and "ASKS FOR HELP", you may assist by administering the shot for the victim.

Epi-pen's come in two doses normally:

- Child dose auto injector of 0.15 mg of weight between 33 and 66 pounds.
- Child dose auto injector of .3 mg of weight more than 66 pounds

Today Epi-pen's come in two-packs. The second dose should only be given if EMS is delayed or after 15 minutes of the first dose.

Knowing the tell-tale signs to treating or recognizing anaphylaxis is:

- Any skin symptom, sign or swollen lips with trouble breathing is anaphylaxis.
- Recognized exposure with combine signs is anaphylaxis.
- Known exposure Known sign is anaphylaxis.

Use Epi-Pen Skill sheet for location.

EPI-PEN

Epinephrines for allergic reactions are commonly found today. The important information is to remember once you decided to inject your victim you follow two simple procedures.

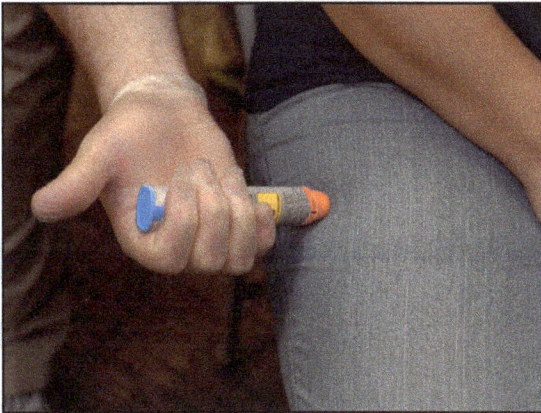

Once you remove it from the package, remove the plastic safety seal cap. Place the orange pointed side down onto the victim thigh area.

This will go through most all material the victim will have on.

Press firmly the blue cap area and hold it.

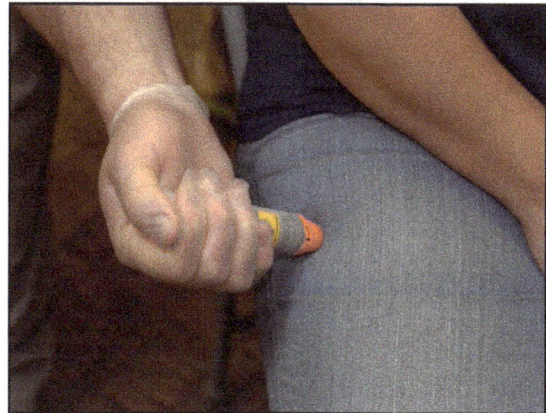

Once you squeeze the injector hold it in place for count of 10 second.

Your victim may not feel any sensation from the shot for 2-3 minutes as its starts to work.

Call Emergency Medical Services immediately.

SHOCK

The primary function of treating for shock is to maintain body temperature. Not being able to handle stress or excitement to an injury causes shock. Choking emergency such as a blocked airway can cause shock from fear or anxiety.

The early onset of shock can be noted by decreased blood flow. Skin can become pale or bluish, cool to touch, clammy, skin moist.

When checking the victim, Pulse may be increased >100. Respirations may increase >30. If a upper body injury has been noticed then breathing will be rapid and shallow.

The victim may hemorrhage becoming restless or excited and complaining of thirst. Upon interviewing the victim, you may determine that a small amount of water in a bottle cap may be given. This will help to calm the victim. If you suspect any form of abdominal injury do not give any amount of fluids.

Late signs of Shock are determined by unresponsiveness. Eyes may become withdraw and a blank expressions and pupils may be large.

Shock is a condition in which there is loss of effective circulating blood volume. Inadequate organ and tissue perfusion results, ultimately causing cellular metabolic derangements. In all emergency situations, it is wise to anticipate shock before it develops. Any injured person should be assessed immediately to determine the presence of shock.

Common Causes of Shock: bleeding, poisoning, insect bites, snake bites, electrical shock, burns, severe injuries, psychological trauma, heart attack, and other medical conditions.

Signs and Symptoms:

- Pale or bluish lips, gums, and fingernails.
- Clammy skin in touch, spotted in color.
- Weakness.
- Hard to breath or irregular gasps. Can include anxiety, thirst, and nausea.

ACTION: FIRST AID

FIRST AID for shock: Keep victim lying still but comfortable. Cover them with a blanket to maintain body temperature. Call EMS/9-1-1

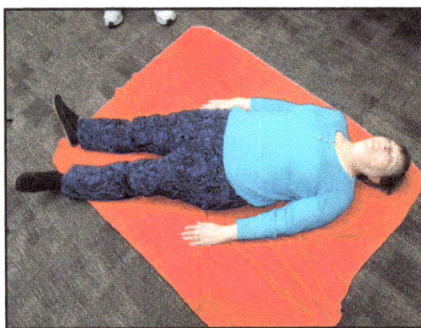

Keep victim lying flat and straight

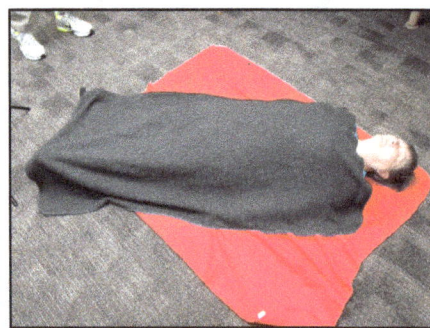

Cover victim with blanket to maintain
core body temperature

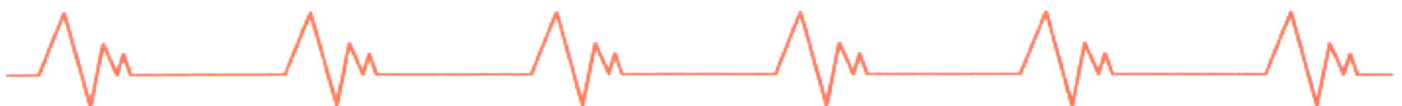

RECOVERY POSITION

This position places your victim on their side in instances when the rescuer has to check on another victim at the scene or get medical help. This allows the victim to breathe easier, maintain and open airway. If you suspect a head, neck or back injuries do not place the victim in this position.

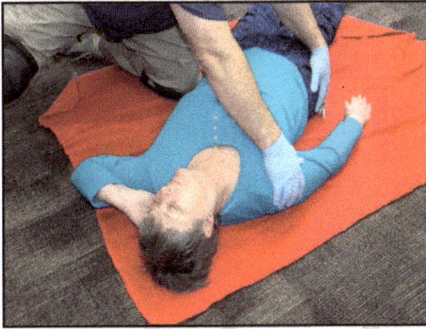

RECOVERY POSISTION

Start placing victims hand near the side of the face. Place your hands, one on the shoulder the other on the hip. Roll your victim towards you. You are positioned close enough to prevent them from rolling flat.

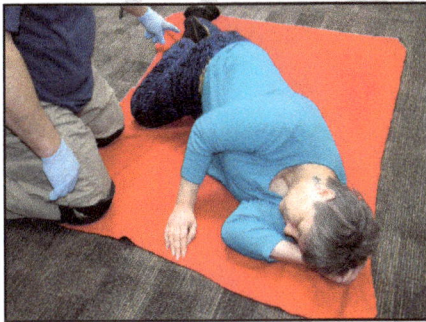

Notice the foot is resting on the lower knee, prompting the upper leg at 45 degree angle to prevent forward motion.

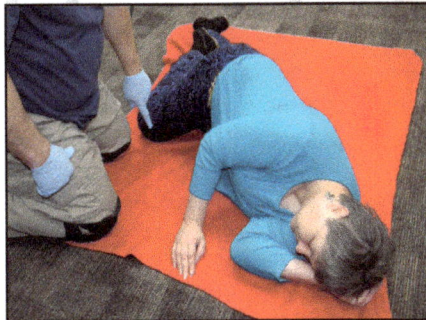

The knee is touching the ground solid to prevent any roll movement.

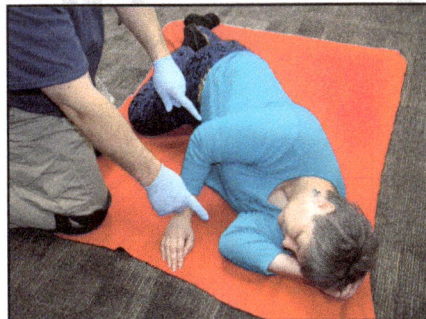

Both elbows are in 45 degree angle positions to prevention movement.

The one arm is bent under the head supports the head and allows for an opening if the victim becomes nauseous.

The victim should never be left alone for any length of period as this is only a temporary position.

BURNS

1st, 2nd, 3rd degree

By definition is an injury from chemicals, heat, radiation or electrical.

Burns by depth determine level of classification:

First, and foremost, on all burns: Submerge all burns in cool tap water for fifteen (15) minutes, then wrap with a moist bandage. KEEP BANDAGE MOIST. Never pop a blister. Treat for shock. Call EMS/9-1-1. Never use butter, margarine, or a petroleum product to cover burned area.

These require minor medical care as soon as possible.

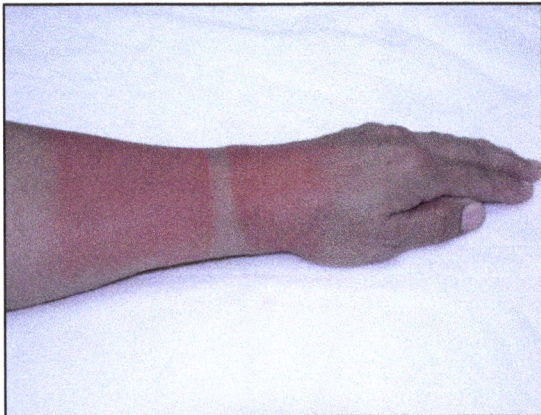

"First degree" burns are usually caused by: Sunburns, touching hot objects lightly, steam, electrical small appliances or hot water, coffee etcetera.

Fast tips for sun burns. Act fast. If you feel the tale-tell tingling of a burn or see any sign of skin reddening on yourself, get out of the sun and start treatment. "Sunburn tends to sneak up on us. It can take four to six hours for the symptoms to develop.

Moisturize and hydrate quickly. Any burn draws fluid to the skin surface and away from the rest of the body. So drink extra water, juice and sports drinks for a couple of days and watch for signs of dehydration: Dry mouth, thirst, reduced urination, headache, dizziness and sleepiness. Anyone with a sunburn who is suffering fevers and chills should also seek medical help,

Take a dose of ibuprofen (for example, Advil) as soon as you see signs of sunburn and keep it up for the next 48 hours, "It cuts back on the swelling and redness that is going to occur" and might prevent some long-term skin damage.

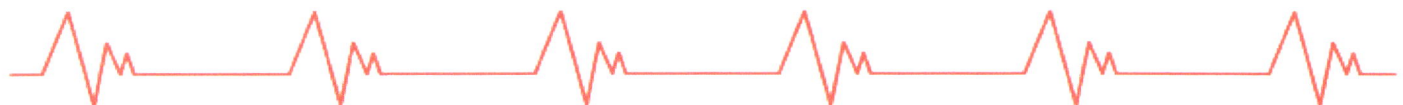

BURNS (CONT'D)

These require immediate moisture over the area by placing a "loose moist towel" over the entire area. Do not apply pressure with the moist towels.

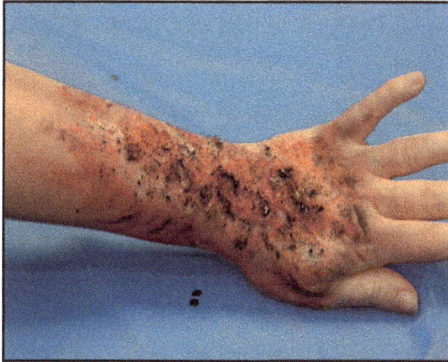

"Second degree" burns are usually caused by: Severe sunburns, extremely hot liquids in contact with the body, flash burns from electricity, flammable fuels. These types of burn penetrate the skin area deeper and are colored by darker reddening of the skin. Blisters can arise and swelling over the area in probable.

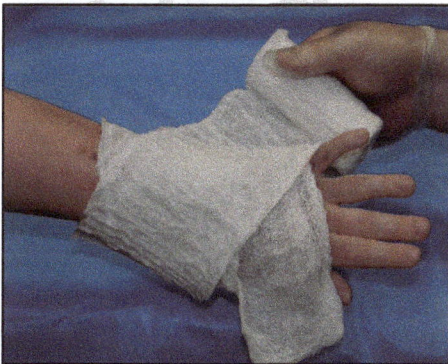

Start with a "loose moist or damp wrap and completely cover the burn lightly. Minimize skin contact as nerve ending have been damaged. Do not apply ointments, creams or jells. "Silverdine" may be recommended after medical help has treated the burn professionally.

"Third degree" burns are usually caused by flames, extreme long period of contact with hot water over 2-3 seconds, flammable liquids, hazardous cleaning fluids or electrical contact. Immediate signs of deep level tissue damage colored by white areas or black charred edges. 100% total destruction of area is imminent. Under thermal conditions anyone suffering burns to any part of the body is critical more important if burns are of the hands, face and upper body immediate hospitalization is required.

First aid action is immediate. Relieving pain, minimizing contact and protecting the area is essential. Never remove charred clothes or material from the area. Immediately cover with light weight cloth and apply moisture to the cloth to prevent air contact or exposure to air. DO NOT USE creams, ointments, butter, grease, mayonnaise no homemade remedies. Get victim to the hospital immediately.

ELECTRICAL SAFETY

Most electrical burns appear to be minor but they can burn "layers" of tissue beneath the skin. Without knowing electrical burns can send shock wave through the body causing internal complications. Cardiac arrest or cardiac-arrhythmia.

If the victim has receive a "jolt" "fallen-down" or thrown by the electrical charge emergency medical attention is immediate.

Keep victim still and comfortable until EMS 9-1-1 arrives. If the heart has stopped begin CPR. Cover the area with dry clean cloth. Do not use fuzzy material as this irritates the area.

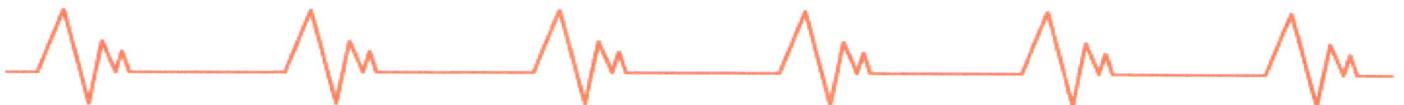

CHEMICAL BURNS

If a toxic or chemical irritant burns the skin:

Place an N95 or greater face breathing barrier on plus chemical proof gloves first.

Remove the cause of the burn by flushing or running water over the area 10 – 15 minutes or until you determine the product has been removed from the area. Remember power chemicals can be brushed off or removed by fanning the area. Please make sure the power chemicals are downwind.

Remove jewelry or clothing that has been contaminated.

Wrap a "dry" cloth or dressing around the area to minimize air contact.

If the victim starts complaining about the burn area rehydrate the area and leave a moist-to wet bandage over the area.

In most case minor chemical burns heal without medical treatment.

Get to the emergency care if the victim has:

ACTION: FIRST AID

- Signs of shock, fainting, become pale or bluish
- Breathing becomes erratic
- Chemical burn area is larger than 2-3 inches with blisters
- If chemical burn is in major organ area, eyes, face, groin, buttocks or joints

In all cases contact the Poison Control Center by dialing 9-1-1 for immediate assistance.

CHEMICAL SPLASH

If a chemical splashes into the eye:

ACTION: FIRST AID

- Flush the eye with water immediately. Use drinking water. Importance is on the diluting of the chemical fast.
- Perform the flushing for 10 – 15 minutes.
- Get emergency help if symptoms such as pain, visual blurring or burning sensation occur.
- Follow treatment directions on the container if located that chemical that burn.

BLISTERS

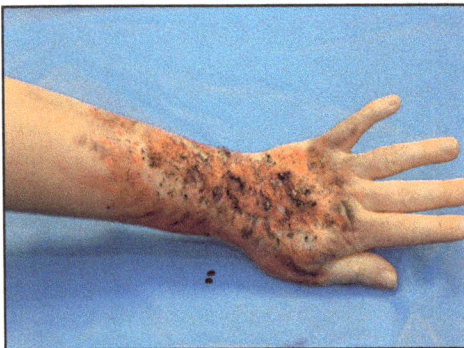

"Blisters" can sometimes be cause by different levels of burns in combination. NEVER pop a blister. Consider the body repairing itself by using blisters. These can be a sign the burned area is topical and the body's defense it to place a balloon of water over the area to heal.

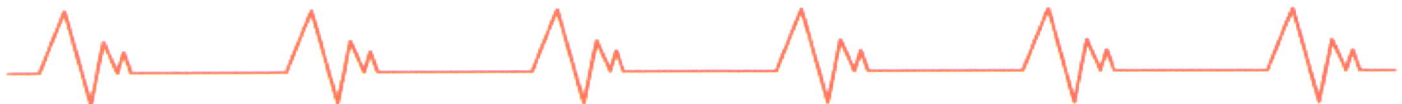

NOSE INJURIES

Severe nose bleeds can be frightening to the victim. It is possible that enough blood can be lost to cause shock.

For nose bleeds: Tip victim's head forward, chin to chest, pinch nose at lowest point. Keep victim calm. IMPORTANT: If you suspect a head, neck, or back injury, DO NOT MOVE THE VICTIM. Keep victim still. It might be necessary to treat for shock.

TOOTH LOSS

When a tooth is accidentally knocked out seek emergency medical care. When permanent tooth/teeth are knocked out sometimes acting fast they can be reimplanted if handled properly.

- Handle tooth by the top side only, NEVER TOUCH THE ROOTS
- Do not try to remove dirt, scrape or rub
- Briefly rinse tooth in normal water, never submerge in running water

BITES AND STINGS

Introduction

Treat all bites serious. The bite could cause one of many reactions including allergic reactions to shock.

When a bite or sting happens, monitoring the victim is essential to maintain open air and observe any signs of allergic reactions.

Human and animal bites are the most common and the most dangerous. Dangerous infection can develop even from a minor bite.

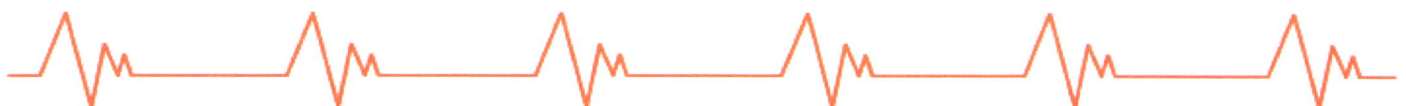

VENOMOUS SNAKES

Venomous snakes cause some 8,000 of the 45,000 snakebites that occur each year in the USA and 9 to 15 deaths per year are attributed to these snakebites. Children between the ages of 1 and 9 years are the most likely victims. The greatest number of bites occurs during daylight hours in summer months. Venomous snakebites are medical emergencies. Call EMS/9-1-1.

Most snakes are not poisonous. A few exceptions include the rattlesnake, coral snake, water moccasin and copperhead.

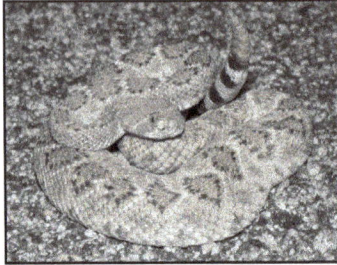

Eastern or western Diamond-back Rattlesnake has two tone skin with brown diamonds running the length of the snake.

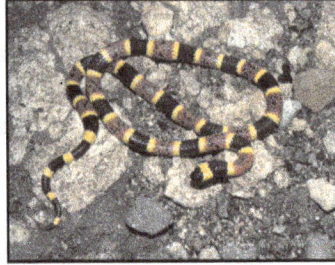

Coral snake can be identified as friend or foe by remembering this simple saying, Red and Black friend of Jack, Red and Yellow killed a fellow.

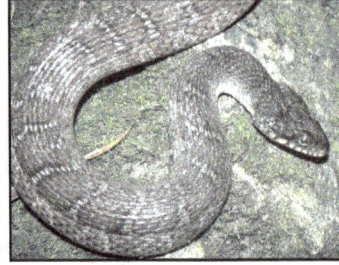

Water moccasin : It is recognized by a brown, olive or blackish dark body with lighter belly, and body crossbands which have a distinct border extending all the way around and across the yellowish stomach.

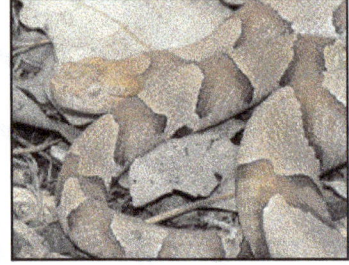

Copperheads are usually colorful and strikingly patterned snakes. The background color of the back and sides is tan to pinkish. There are darker, chestnut colored bands across the back and sides. Each hourglass shaped band is of varying width.

ACTION: FIRST AID

- Call 9-1-1 Immediately.
- Treat for Shock - keep the victim calm (to keep from pumping the poison to other parts of the body).
- Keep victim warm.
- Remove all constrictive items such as rings.
- Immobilize the bitten area and keep it lower than the heart.
- Apply a clean bandage on the area to minimize the contamination any further.
- Do NOT place ice or a tourniquet on the area (as it may speed up the poison by causing shock).
- Monitor the victim's C, A, B's.
- Get medical help as soon as practicable.
- If you can identify the snake poisonous / non-poisonous advise EMS/9-1-1 or the hospital of its type for antivenin purposes.
- Do NOT attempt or allow the victim to drive a car, even to a hospital.
- If you suspect that your pet has been bitten by a snake, keep the animal calm - carry to the car if possible, and dive to the veterinarian's.

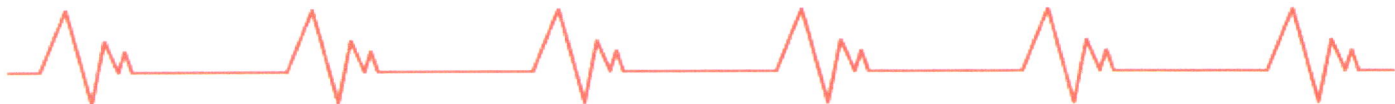

ANIMAL BITES

Domestic animals cause most bite injuries. Leading the numbers are dogs with cats running second place. Cat bites are more likely to cause reactions and infections. Non-vaccinated pets run a risk of carrying Rabies. Rabies are found in skunks, raccoons, foxes, bats, possums. Rarely rabbits, squirrels are infected. If you suspect someone has been bitten by and animal with rabies:

ACTION: FIRST AID

1. If the bite breaks the skin treat the wound as a minor injury. Wash thoroughly. If available apply an antibiotic cream and cover the area.
2. If the bitten area has torn skin treat as open wound, apply direct pressure, wrap.
3. If redness or swelling is notice get medical help immediately.
4. If any animal bite is suspected of an non-immunized animal seek medical help immediately.

Department of Health guidelines "suggest" a recommendation of a tetanus shot every 10 years. If you cannot remember when your last tetanus shot was given then have a new shot. In some instances doctors may require a "booster" shot within 2 days.

INSECT BITES AND STINGS

Most symptoms of an insect bite result from the injection of venom or other defense agent into the skin. The venom triggers an allergic reaction. The reaction depends on each person immune system.

Majority of reactions are mild causing an annoying sensation or itch which will go away in a day or two. Some reactions may cause shortness of breath, swelling, hives, swollen glands and pain in joints.

Small insects, bees, wasps, hornets, yellow jackets, biting flies, spiders, mosquitoes or fire ants are typically the most annoying.

When Mild Reactions occur:

- Move to a safe location
- Remove the stinger
- Place ice (in plastic bag if available)
- If victim is NOT allergic place hydrocortisone, calamine lotion on the area.
- Victim may take an Antihistamine or Benadryl

When Severe Reactions occur:

Call 9-1-1 if:
- Difficulty breathing
- Swelling in the mouth. Lips or throat
- Faint
- Rapid or accelerated heart beat
- Hives
- Confusion
- Nausea, cramping or regurgitating (vomiting)

Until 9-1-1 arrives:
- Have the victim lie down
- If unconscious place victim in the Recovery Position to expel liquids from the mouth
- If a victim stops breathing begin CPR
- Look on the victim's person or property for allergy kit (epinephrine)

For bites and stings: Wash off all bites with soap and water to prevent allergic reaction. Place ice over the area to prevent swelling.

INSECT BITES AND STINGS (CONT'D)

Insect Bites and Stings: Ants, bees, wasps, spiders, etc. - Use a dull flat surface to gently move upward and downward on stinger area to remove stinger. Do not use tweezers as this may cause further infection.

Spiders: Seek immediate medical help for bites from Black Widow or Brown Recluse or Scorpions. Treat for shock immediately.

How to Remove a Bee Stinger

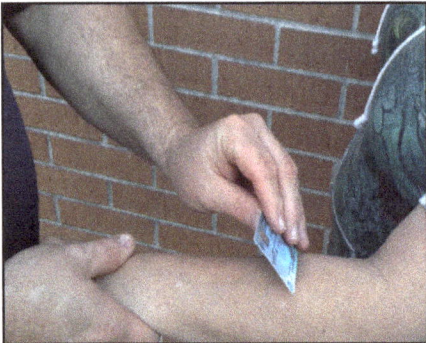

Use Credit card or hard thin card to start above the bitten area

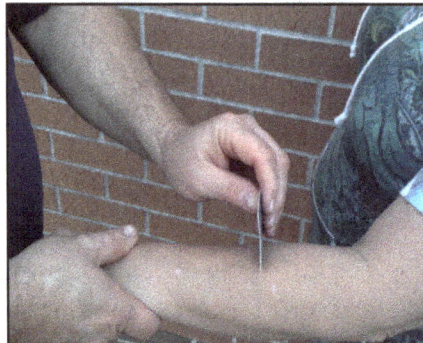

Scrape and drag Pull down across the stinger area

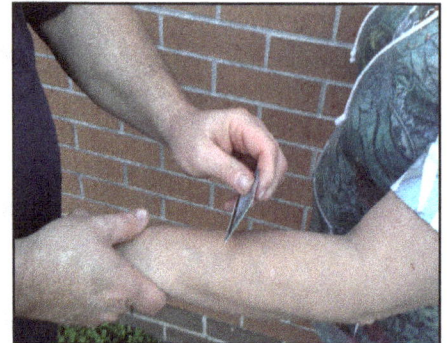

Finish by lifting credit card in a curving sweep motion to life stinger off skin

Once you have removed the stinger place a "single ice-cube" over the area to help relieve any swelling. Then dry off and cover with bandage. Watch victim for allergic reactions.

TICK BITES

Many Ticks transmit bacteria that cause illnesses like Lyme disease or Rocky Mountain spotted fever. If precautions are taken, and what part of the United States you live, how much outdoor activity you perform and how much time you spend with animals that carry ticks.

If you're bitten by a tick and it embeds itself into you, try the following:

Ticks are breathers, they need oxygen to survive. Simple extraction techniques vary from using tweezers at the base of the tick closest to the skin and lightly squeezing the tick to remove. Other techniques may require you to simply limit the air around the tick by using oil around and over the area. This will encourage the tick to "back-out" without leaving any parts in the skin.

ACTION: FIRST AID

You must get medical attention if you see signs of:
- Rash
- Fever
- Muscle Aches
- Joint pain or swelling

Remember to take the tick in a plastic bag with you to the emergency care. This will help to identify the treatment faster.

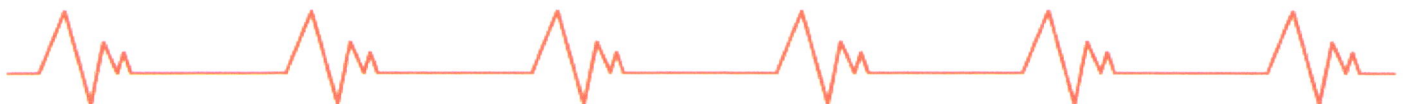

SPIDER BITES

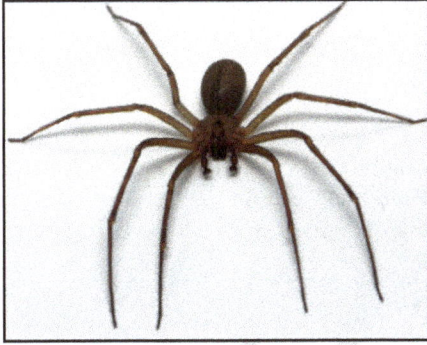

BROWN RECLUSE SPIDER

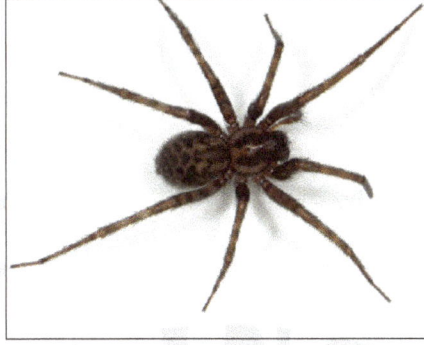

WOLFE SPIDER

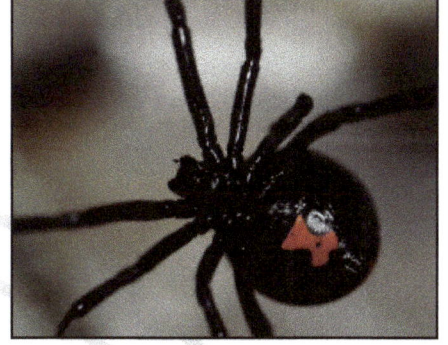

BLACK WIDOW SPIDER

Brown Recluse

Brown recluse spiders are native to the Midwestern and Southeastern states. Documented populations of brown recluse spiders outside these areas are extremely rare.

Wolfe Spider

Wolf spiders live almost everywhere in the world, they are especially common in grasslands and meadows, but also live in mountains, deserts, rainforests and wetlands — anywhere they can find insects to eat.

Black widow

The female black widow has unusually large venom glands and her bite is particularly harmful to humans; however notorious, bites are rarely fatal.

HUMAN BITES

is the skin broken? Immediate care for human bites is a simple washing the area off. Use plain soap and water. Using other styles of cleaning could lead to or accelerate the allergic reaction. When a bite or sting happens monitoring the victim is essential to maintain open air and observe any signs of allergic reactions. Treatments for allergic reactions can have several options. Using and EpiPen, (Epinephrine).

Human and animal bites are the most common and the most dangerous. Dangerous infection can develop even from a minor bite. Prevent infection by either wearing latex gloves or first wash your hands. If bleeding is not severe, wash wound with soap and water, cover with a clean dressing. Watch for allergic reaction. Treat all bites serious. The bite could cause any of the following reactions, from allergic reactions to shock.

Most infants and young children bite occasionally. Usually a bite is harmless and may not even leave a mark. Infants most often bite in response to new sensations in the mouth, such as may occur when teething. Young children may bite out of frustration because they cannot yet translate their emotions into words.

ACTION: FIRST AID

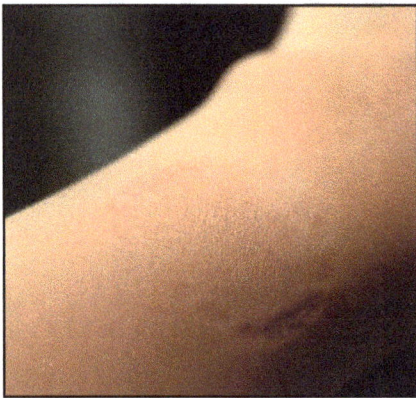

A minor human bite is one where the skin has not been punctured or if the skin has been broken, bleeding and tissue damage are not severe.

First

- Wash the bitten area thoroughly. Use running water and soap
- Apply pressure with a clean dry cloth to bites where the skin has been broken in order to stop any bleeding
- Dress the bitten area with gauze or sterile dressing. This is a preventative measure to keep the area clean and infection-free

Bites on children: Wash bitten area thoroughly with soap and water. DO NOT use antiseptic, ointments or other medications. These may cause an allergic reaction. Put a single ice cube on the area to prevent swelling. Document all bite cases.

Call 911 if:

- A human bite causes serious injury.
- The wound will not stop bleeding after 10 minutes of firm pressure.
- Blood spurts from the wound.

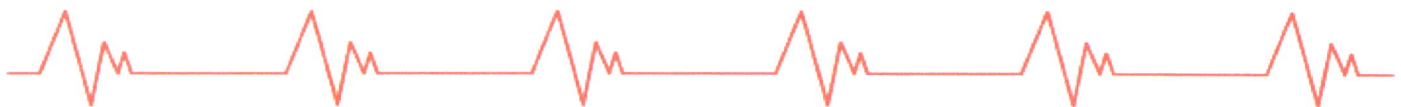

POISONING

Vector, Swallowed, Inhalation, Absorption

A poison is any substance; solid, liquid, or gas, that causes injury or death when introduced into the body. There are four (4) main ways a person can be poisoned; by inhaling, absorbing, injecting, and/or swallowing.

IN ALL CASES CALL EMS/9-1-1.

You must have permission before administering Syrup of Ipecac; NEVER give this to infants (anyone under 18 months of age). NEVER give this without permission from the doctor. Never dilute without permission from a doctor. Keep a sample of any vomit. Keep all containers from the poison. Never induce vomiting if you see blisters. The most common mistake is people calling the information number in an emergency. The emergency number for poisoning is EMS/9-1-1.

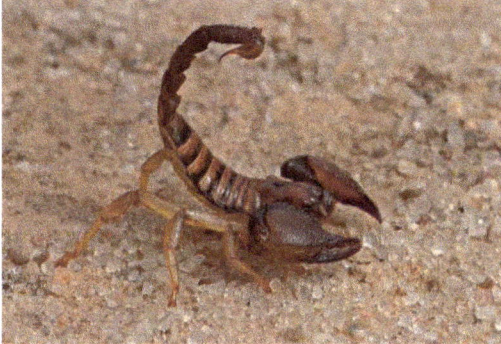

Scorpions can hide in places and blend in like camouflage. When your cleaning or moving boxes, storage material they will be there when you least expect them.

ACTION: FIRST AID

For Snake bites: Keep the victim calm. Remove all constrictive items such as rings. Keep victim warm. Keep the bitten area below the level of the heart. Apply a clean bandage on the area to minimize the contamination any further. Do NOT place ice or a tourniquet on the area. This may speed up the poison by causing shock. Monitor the victim's C, A, B's. Get help immediately. If you can identify the snake poisonous / non-poisonous advise EMS/9-1-1 or the hospital of its type for antivenin purposes.

DIABETIC EMERGENCY

Hypoglycemia versus Hyperglycemia

Generally a person who is Diabetic can range in numbers for Hypo vs. Hyper.

Blood sugars numbers varies but for the average test numbers from 100 – 130 are normal.

Hypoglycemia means sugars are LOW and the person needs to eat to bring numbers up.

Hyperglycemia means sugars are HIGH and need insulin injection to bring the numbers down.

This is when a person has taken medication but has not eaten. HYPOGLYCEMIA Signs and Symptoms: Moist, pale, clammy skin. Profuse cold sweat. May include: hunger, shortness or shallow breathing, confusion, trembling hands, shaking, weakness, dizziness and personality change.

ACTION: FIRST AID

For Hypoglycemia: Give the victim something containing sugar, orange juice, candy, or sugar in any form if they are conscious. This should bring improvements within a few minutes. If this does not bring a change within a few minutes Call EMS/9-1-1.

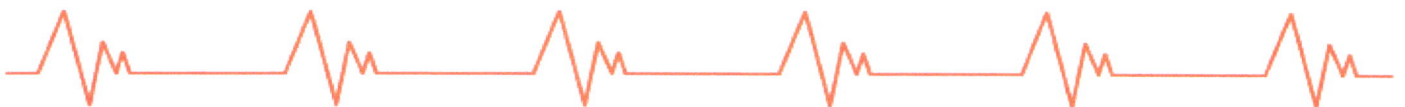

HEAT STROKE VS. HEAT EXHAUSTION

Heatstroke

On hot, humid days with no breeze, anyone may be affected by the heat. They may suffer heat stroke, heat exhaustion, or heat cramps. The body temperature can rise so high that brain damage and death may result if the body is not quickly cooled down. Quickly cool the victim's body. Heat stroke requires medical attention.

Signs and Symptoms of **Heatstroke**:

Hot, red skin, very small pupils, and very high body temperature sometimes as high as 105° degrees. Rapid pulse. Confusion or disorientation. Unconsciousness. (Hot, red raise the head)

ACTION: FIRST AID

Call EMS/9-1-1. Get the person out of the heat and into a cooler place. Immerse him or her in a cool bath, wrap wet sheets around the body and fan it. Reduce temperature to 101° degrees. Give nothing by mouth. Do not give medications.

Heat Exhaustion

Heat Exhaustion is less dangerous than heat stroke. Fluid loss causes blood flow to decrease in the vital organs, resulting in a form of shock. With heat exhaustion, sweat does not evaporate as it should, possibly because of high humidity or too many layers of clothing. As a result, the body is not cooled effectively. (Cool, pale raise the tail)

Signs and Symptoms of **Heat Exhaustion**:

Cool, pale, and moist skin – heavy sweating, dilated pupils, headache, nausea, dizziness, and vomiting. Body temperature will be nearly normal. (Cool and pale raise the tail)

ACTION: FIRST AID

Get the person out of the heat. Place him or her in the shock position, remove or loosen the victim's clothing. Cool him or her by fanning and applying cold packs. Use wet towels or sheets. Give the victim ½ glassful of water to drink every 15 minutes, if he or she is fully conscious. These steps should bring improvement within a half hour.

HEAT CRAMPS

Most Heat cramps are painful and involuntarily muscle spasms. Common during heavy lifting, exercising. Dehydration is common. Areas of cramps include arms, legs, thighs, calves, abdomen back and hands. Common mistakes are induced salt tablets and lack of hydration induces cramps.

ACTION: FIRST AID

- Rest briefly and cool down.
- Induce liquids containing electrolytes.
- Before engaging exercise, stretch or extend muscles.

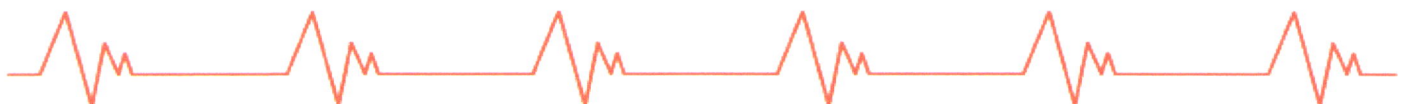

FROSTBITE

When long periods of exposure to very cold temperatures the skin tissues may freeze, resulting in frostbite. Common areas affected are ears, nose, fingers, hands and feet. Frostbite starts by discoloration, lite grayish to pale skin. Lite frostbite the skin can become red and painful.

ACTION: FIRST AID

- Immediately get out of the cold.
- Cover affected areas.
- Do NOT RUB affected areas.
- Do NOT induce alcohol.
- Room temperature water may be use, NO HOT WATER

HYPOTHERMIA

Normally the human body maintains a safe temperature. When exposed to cold temperatures or extreme cool environment for long periods your body fails to maintain a normal temperature.

If someone has fallen in cold water or outside in extreme cold wet environments increase hypothermia.

Hypothermia happens when the body's core temperature falls below 94 degrees. Immediate tell tale signs are:

- Shivering
- Slurred speech
- Reduced breathing, slower than normal
- Cold, cool pale skin
- Loss of balance or coordination
- Slow to react, fatigue or lethargic

Hypothermia happens over a gradual period of time. Victims often lose mental alertness or ability to physically move.

ACTION: FIRST AID

- Remove the victim out of the cold
- Insulate the body and head immediately
- Remove wet clothing, place dry clothes on the victim
- Watch the victims breathing and monitor pulse every 2 minutes
- Never induce alcohol
- If not regurgitating offer a warm drink not hot

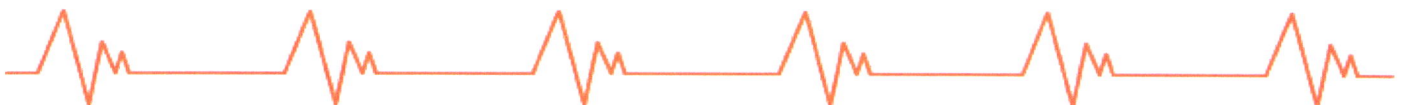

SEIZURES

Seizures may be caused by a temporary problem, insulin shock, high fever, viral infection of the brain, head-neck injury, or drug reactions. Epilepsy is usually well controlled with medication, but some people who have it continue to have seizures from time to time. Some individuals have an aura (sensation) before the onset of a seizure. Auras can be sound and vision hallucinations, a strange taste in the mouth, abdominal pain, numbness, or a sense of urgency to move to safety.

Call EMS/9-1-1 if the victim: has multiple seizures, has never had a seizure before, is pregnant, is diabetic, has swallowed a large amount of water, or has a head injury.

In most cases EMS/9-1-1 does not need to be called: if the victim has been diagnosed with seizures, but do the following:

ACTION: FIRST AID

1. Clear the area to prevent further injury; protect the head, use hands under victim's head, let the victim go completely through the seizure(s), NEVER PUT ANYTHING IN THE MOUTH OF THE VICTIM.

2. Open airway after the seizure(s) stop to check A, B, C's, if not breathing begin CPR. Keep the victim calm.

FRACTURES, SPRAINS, STRAINS, & DISLOCATIONS

As a non-professional, treat all fractures, sprains, and strains as broken limbs. Splint if in doubt. With all suspected fractures it is important to get medical help as fast as possible.

The basic types of musculoskeletal injuries are known to inflict the most pain.

For Fractures: IMPORTANT

ACTION: FIRST AID

Do not move the fractured area. Simply splint the break exactly as you find it. Use magazines, rolled up newspapers, or soft bound books to roll around the suspected area. Tie articles above and below the area for immobilization. Treat for shock. Call EMS/9-1-1.

For Sprain/Strain

ACTION: FIRST AID

Place ice on the area. IMPORTANT – Never place ice directly on the body. Place ice in wet towel or cloth. In case of injury to the feet: leave shoes on: they act as a splint to help keep pressure on the area and to keep injury from swelling. Not all fractures and breaks are noticed with the eyes, please splint even if you suspect a fracture.

By definition are commonly caused by vehicle accidents, recreational activities, slips, trips and falls. Older persons who fall break or dislocate the bones more often as bones become more brittle.

Signs and Symptoms.

In auto accidents persons who are responsiveness can detail the area of injury. Common sounds or positions when the accident occurred.

- They heard or felt a snap or pop sound in the bone
- They may point of help locate the pain, tender area or can't move the area
- They can describe any unusual sounds, grinding, snapping or popping
- They may be able to show where they cannot move the body part.

Always look for signs of bruising, discoloration, body area not normal alignment.

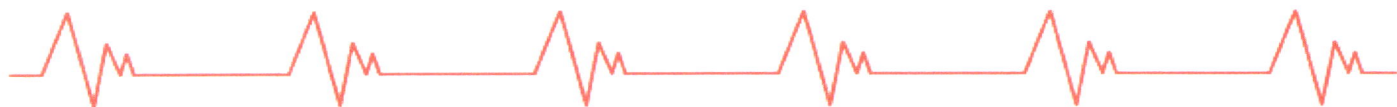

OPEN FRACTURES

The most common "open fractures" include bleeding wounds. Common are bent, distorted or unusual disfigurements. Tissue damage is possible.

CLOSED FRACTURES

The majority of fractures are closed, unable to see the joint injury clearly. When treating these types of injuries all treat with care.

ACTION: FIRST AID

Always immobilize the area above and below the suspected area. When available have the victim seen immediately by an emergency room that can x-ray the area.

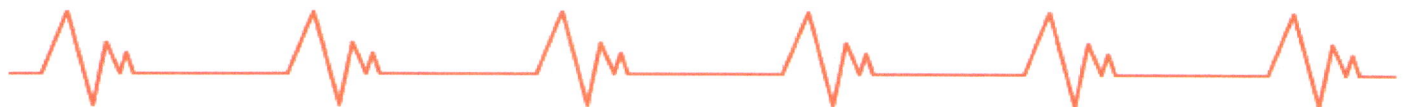

SPLINTING "OPEN OR CLOSED FRACTURE"

The "KEY" of splinting is:

- Reduce pain
- Reduce further damage to the area
- Reduce bleeding
- Reduce loss of use to the area or limb
- Reduce the injury from worse

First use a soft padded firm splint. Use cardboard with a towel or paper towels layer on it to place against the suspected fractured area.

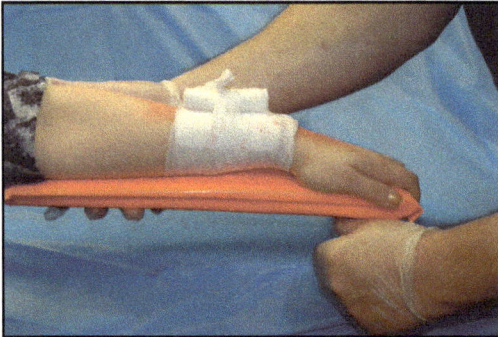

FOREARM SPLINT

First after the area is treated, minor cuts or bleeding place a splint under the area.

Notice the splint stops at her fingers, so you can check color for blood flow.

Extend the splint past her elbow.

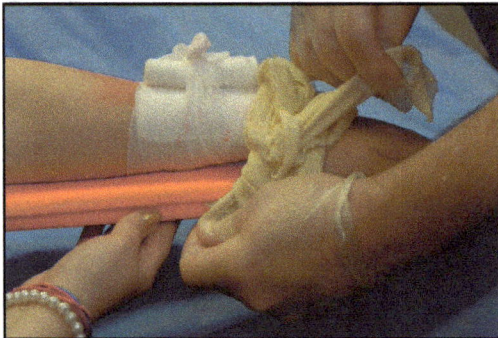

Have victim help to hold splint in place briefly while you place a bandage below the break area.

Notice the bandage is being tied off to the side of the arm between the padded splint and arm. This will allow a pinch free area not causing discomfort to the victim.

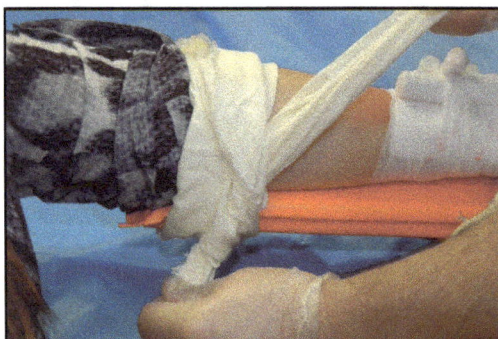

Above the suspected area the second bandage is also tied between the padding and the arm not to cause discomfort.

If you find any loose ends to the tying material tuck this into the padded area.

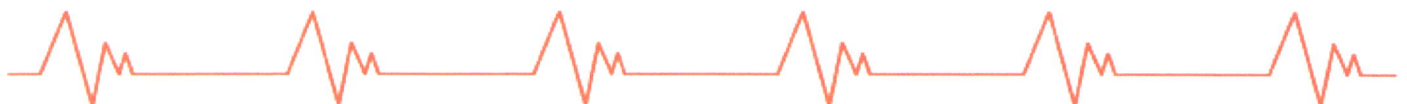

SPRAINS

Commonly known as "twisted knees" "sprained ankles". The body has been forced in different directions and caused a "torn ligament".

When splinting or applying a soft splint as in twisted ankles, remember to "ice" the area until the splint is in place.

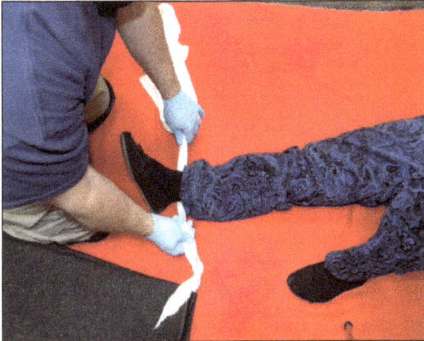

ANKLE SPLINT

Always leave the victims shoes on. This helps to reduce swelling.

Start by sliding under the ankle a bandage.

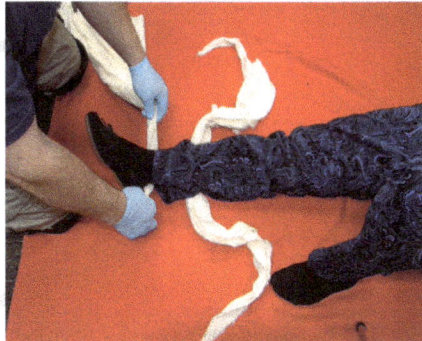

Slide the first bandage up to the lower calf.

Slide a second bandage under the ankle

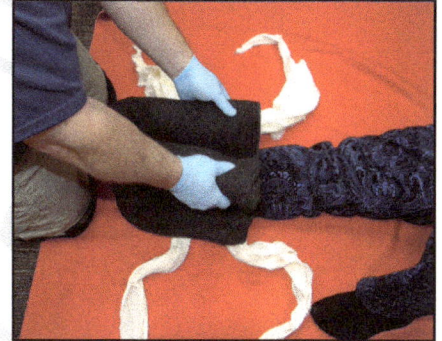

Apply soft blanket or towels around the injured area.

This protects the area while giving support.

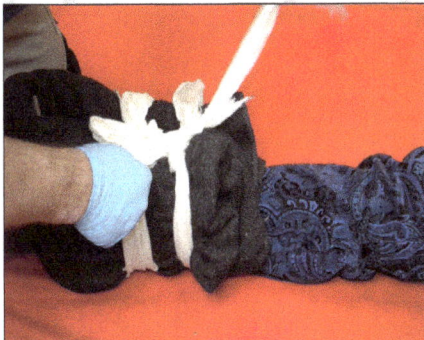

Tie both bandages one above the ankle and the other on the lower calf area.

The knots should be ties using a "double twist" or "double half-hitch" to secure bandage from loosening.

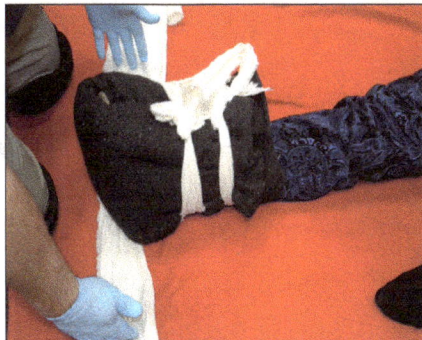

Finishes by applying a "third" bandage hooked around the lower heal of the foot.

This supports the "soft splint".

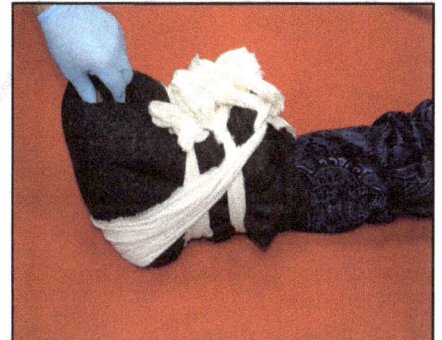

After tying the bandage make sure you can see, feel and touch the tip of the foot.

This can determine blood circulation.

Do not move the victim until proper rescue equipment has arrived.

LEG SPLINTS

Leg splints are important when suspecting a fracture, sprain or strain in a lower major joint. Rescuers are usually alone and have to immobilize the victim fast to prevent further injury. Protecting the injured area is critical for long term care.

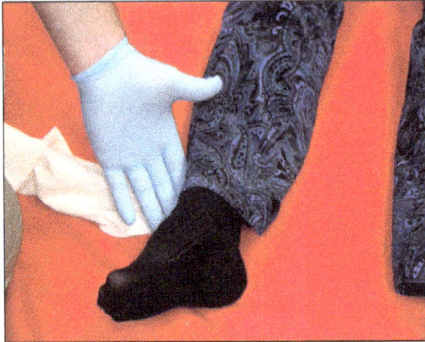

Start by securing bandages under the victim's leg. The lower bandages should be placed on the lower side just above the heel behind the ankle. The body has a natural curve here and you can prevent unnecessary moving the suspected injured are. Place the tip of the first bandage on your finger and slide your finger under the leg pushing bandage across.

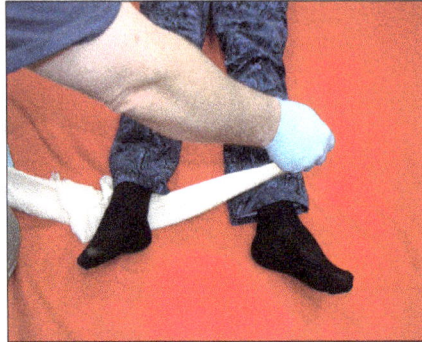

After securing bandaging across victim place almost half on one side.

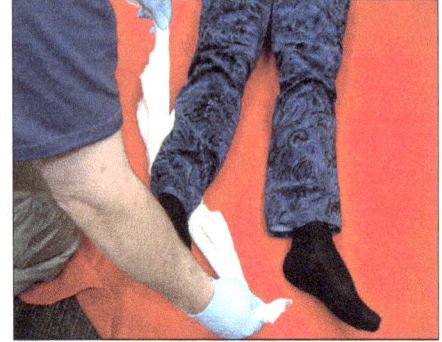

Turn bandage at angle to work bandage up half way on lower calf.

Work the bandage in a sawing motion to slide in under the calf area.

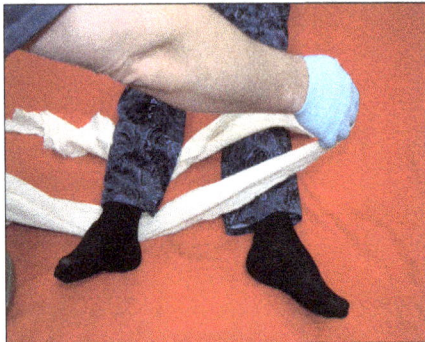

Now you have two bandages on the lower leg.

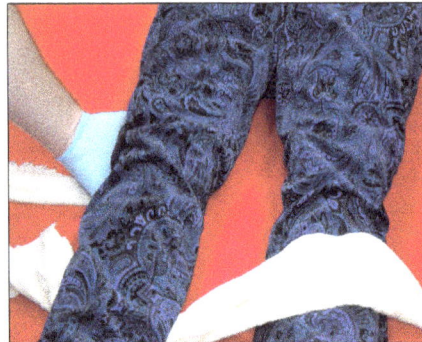

Repeat this process of starting bandages behind the lower knee.

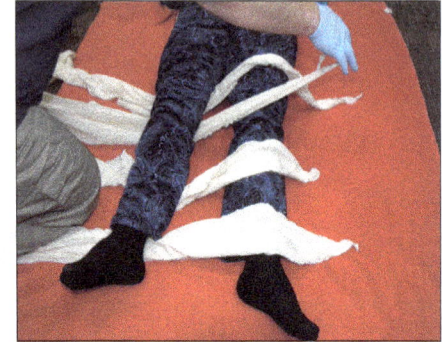

4 bandages are now in place to support the full length leg splint.

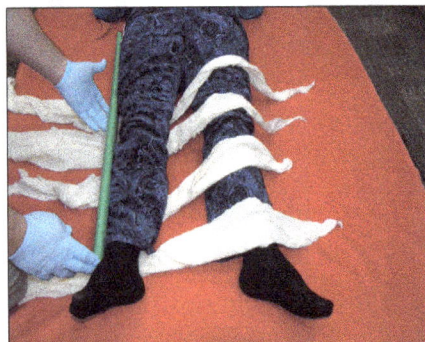

Place splint on outside of leg. This will not interfere with extremities allowing the lower unit to move a one solid unit.

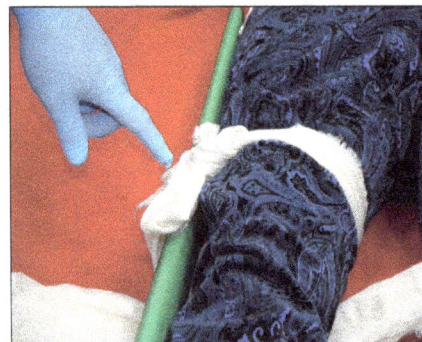

Tying the knot off to the side over the edge of the splint and NOT on the skin helps to prevent further discomfort to the victim.

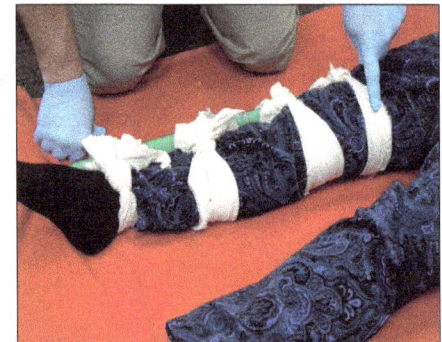

Notice all 4 bandages are securing the splint and the victim to immobilize the fracture, sprain or strain from movement until emergency medical helps arrives.

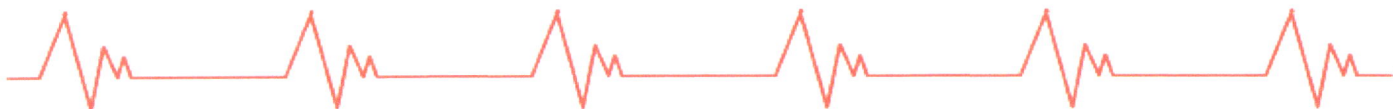

USING AN ARM SLING

Arm sling can be used to help transport a victim with an upward suspected Open or Closed fracture.

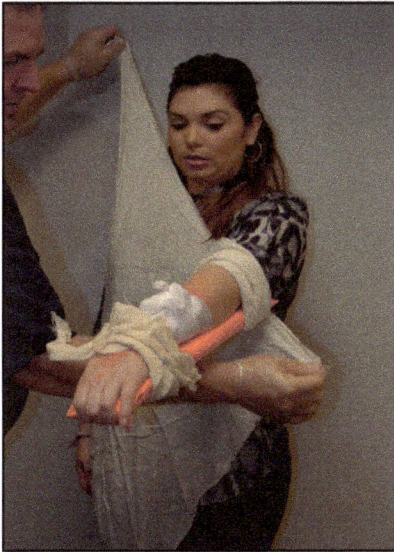

ARM SLING

Establishing the direction of the Arm Sling begins with the "short point" pointing the elbow of the injured arm.

The "2 long points" are placed on the "opposite side of the arm running the length of the body.

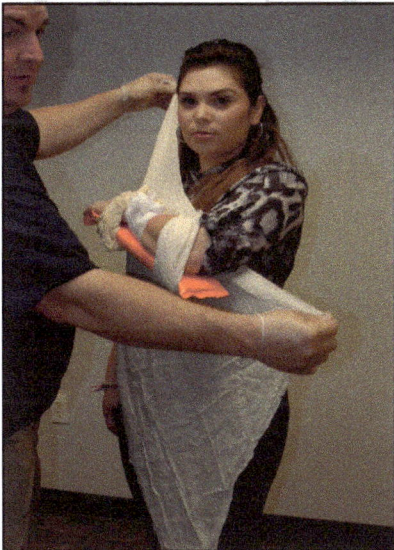

After the forearm sling is tied off secure the short point end by folding the point into the sling. You may "pin" or "tie" this

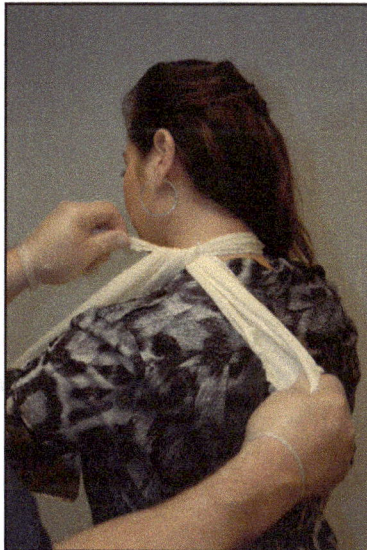

Be sure to tie the knot off on the injured arm side of the neck, This will help to alleviate pain from the arm sling.

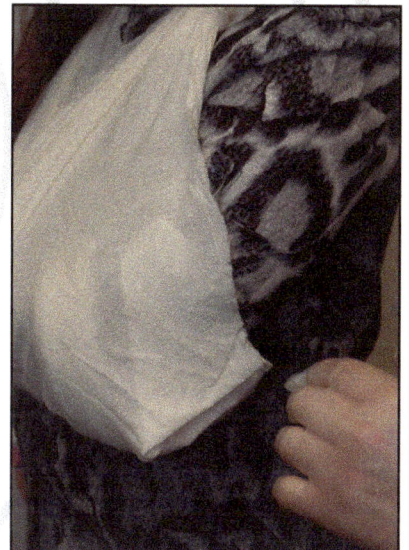

Have the victim move the arm onto the chest area placing the suspected fracture area above the heart. This will minimize "throbbing pain" and offer immediate temporary relief.

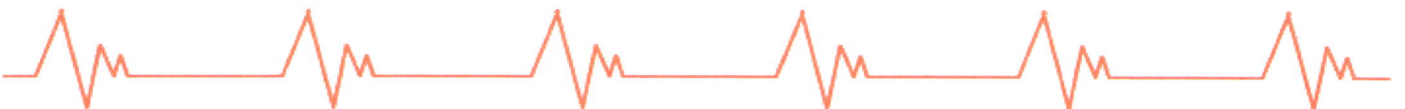

DISLOCATIONS

Dislocations are when bones are out of the normal positions. Often this happens after a fall or hit. Many sports related dislocations are by blunt trauma. Hips, knees, shoulder, elbows, ankles are most common. In almost every dislocation medical attention is required immediately.

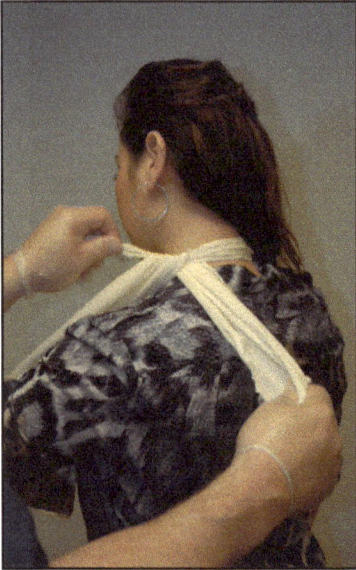

Securing suspected collar bone or shoulder dislocation requires immediate immobilization. When placing triangle bandage around neck area to support the arm make sure the knot is tie off to the side of the neck.

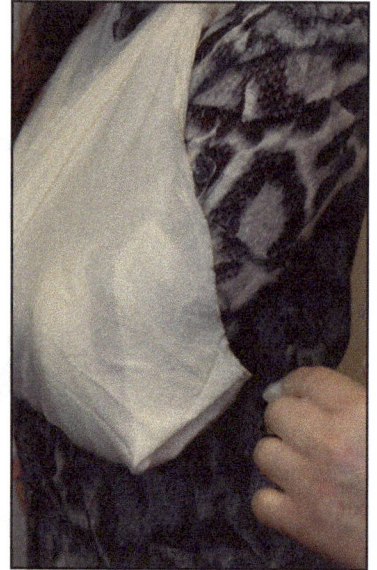

Once bandage is securely tied off enclosed the end on the elbow to keep area from slipping out of bandage.

ACTION: FIRST AID

- Immediately immobilize the area. Use an arm sling to stabilize the area of the shoulder. Hips, knees, ankles use the leg splint.
- Immediate trained medical help can reposition the dislocation is most cases. Rarely does surgery have to be performed.
- Place ice on the area.
- Keep victim calm and still.

ANATOMICAL SPLINTS

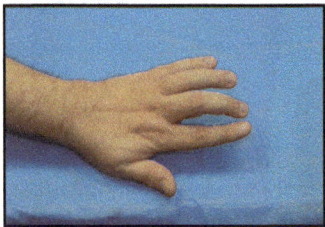

Sprained or Fractured fingers can be used to support each other

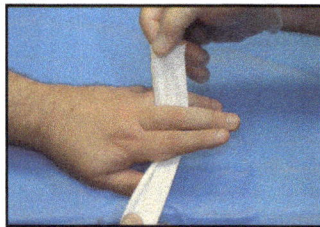

Place tape as close to hand area for greater support

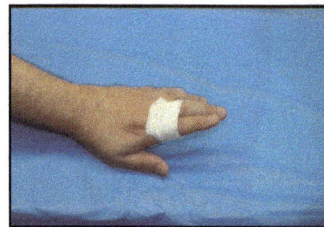

After wrapping lower area apply to upper area

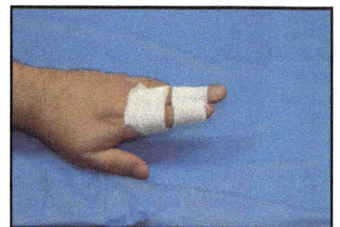

Fingers can now be supported and always follow up with Hospital care

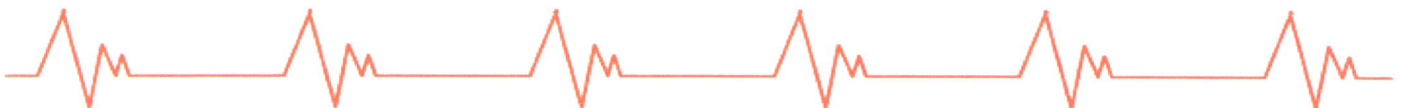

HEAD TRAUMA

The majority of head trauma injuries are minor. Always call 9-1-1 when severe bleeding of the head or face occurs or any changes of consciousness. Black and blues areas around eyes or ears.

- If Head trauma is suspected have victim lie down or sit comfortably still.
- Do not move the neck or head.
- If victim becomes unconscious maintain open airway until emergency helps arrives.

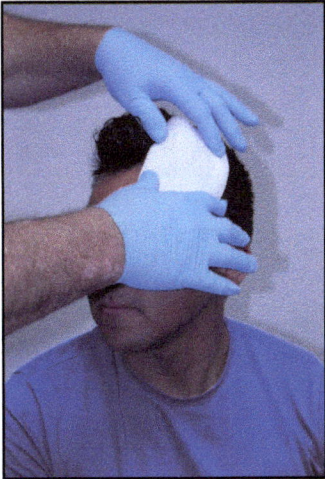

Secure bandage over wound area.

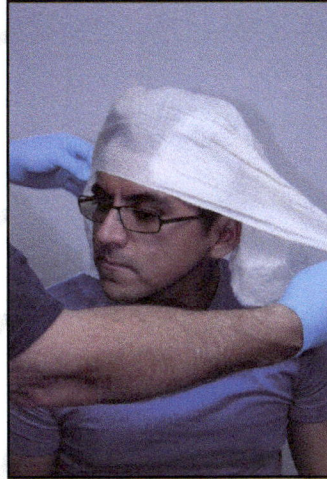

Place Cravat or Triangular bandage over the wound area. Secure the bandage starts just above the eye brows.

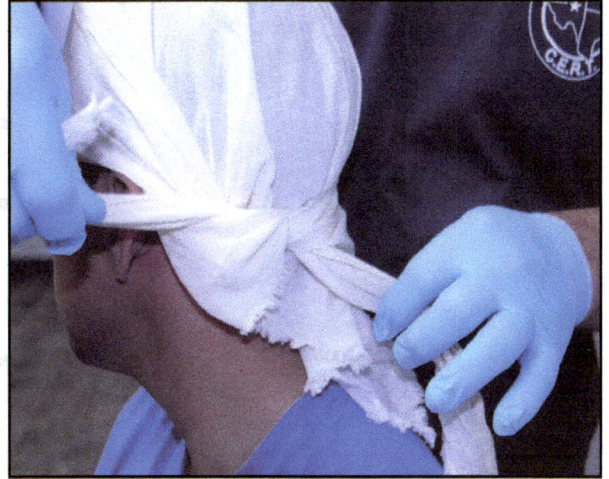

Secure the knot on the side of the neck-head area. NEVER place the knot in back or front of the bandage. If the victim has to be treated for shock this could interfere with the wound area.

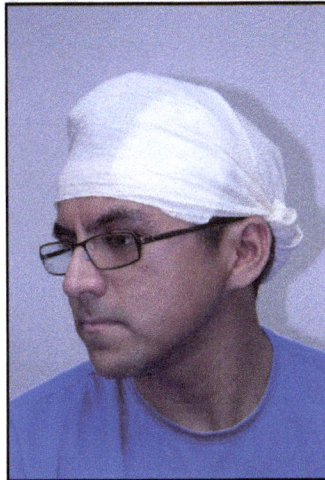

Close the bandage by tucking end the loose ends rolled back into the triangle bandage.

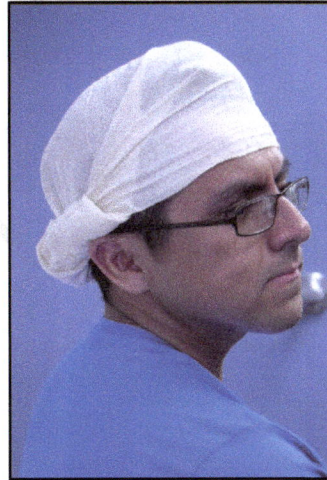

Securing bandage all around help to prevent loose ends from getting pulled or snagged.

2-PERSON HAND CARRY

In certain situations it is extremely important to remove persons with limited mobility. The 2 Person Hand carry is the simplest and easiest to perform.

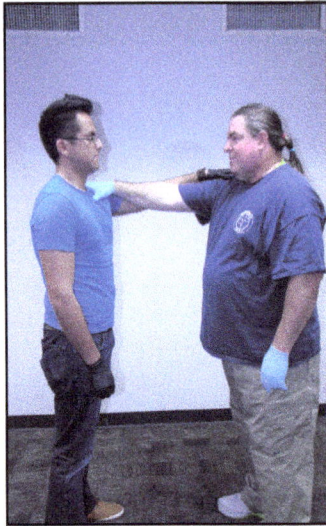

Rescuers turn and face eachother. They place one hand on each other shoul-

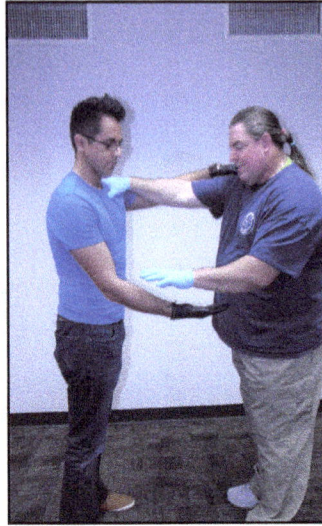

Next they place each others hand out to the front and look at how they will secure their hands together, inter-

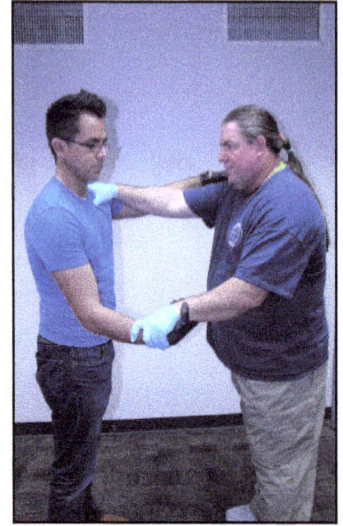

Again they place each other's hand in shoulder location. This time placing each hand with wrist interlocking.

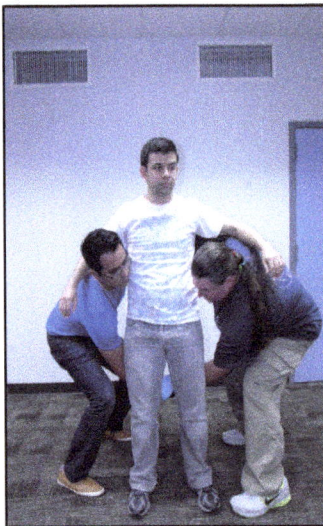

Victim places their arms over each rescuers shoulder. Both rescuers lean over to "scoop" victim up in a "seated position"

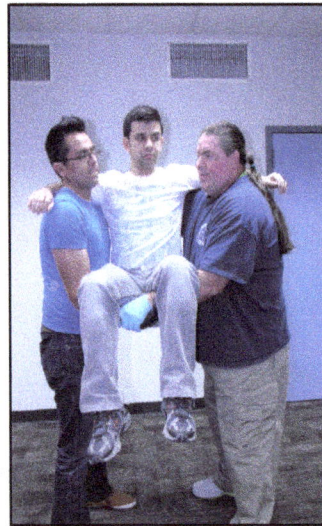

Victim is supported by rescuers. Notice in middle of picture both rescuers hands are interlocked under the knees supporting the victim

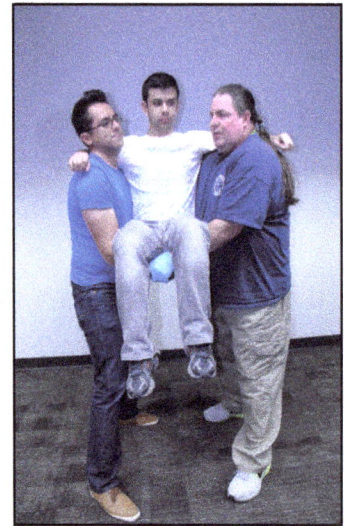

Once victim is stabilized both rescuers start off on with foot in front, left side of victim rescuers starts with left foot, right side of victim rescuers starts off with right foot. This prevents "rocking motion" as victim is moved.

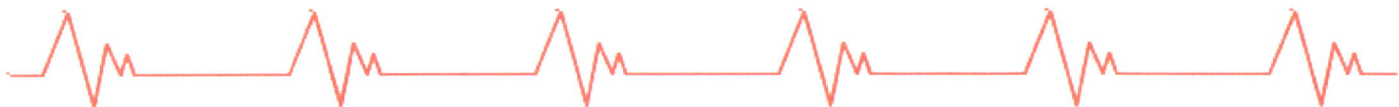

C-SPINE AND IMMOBILIZATION

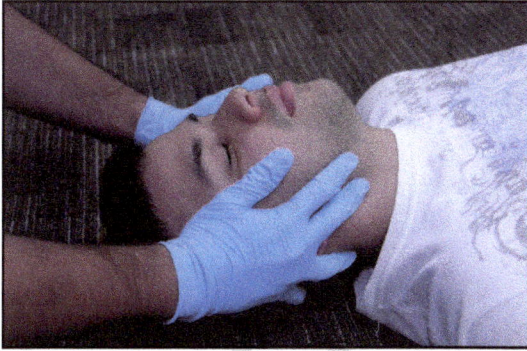

The Term "Hold C-Spine" places emphasis on securing the head-neck stay in-line with the body. This is performed using a modified jaw-thrust. 2 fingers run with the jaw line. 2 more fingers hold just under the ears to the neck to assure head doesn't move.

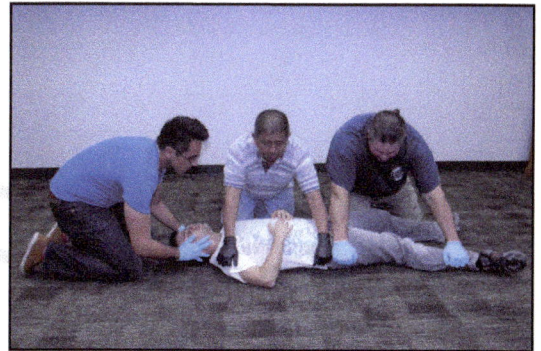

Preparing a victim with c-spine injury requires extra rescuers to roll-victim in a single unit-log. 1 rescuer hold shoulder and hip. 2nd rescuer hold hip and lower legs firmly.

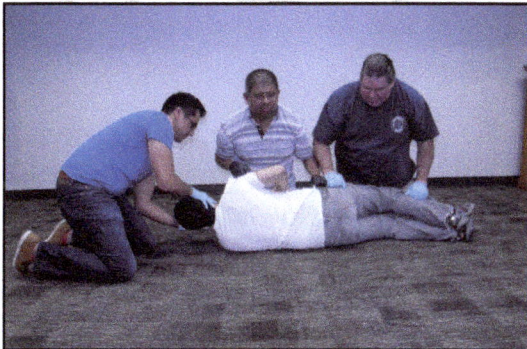

C-spine Rescuer rolls victim head with body as rescuers roll victim to 90º.

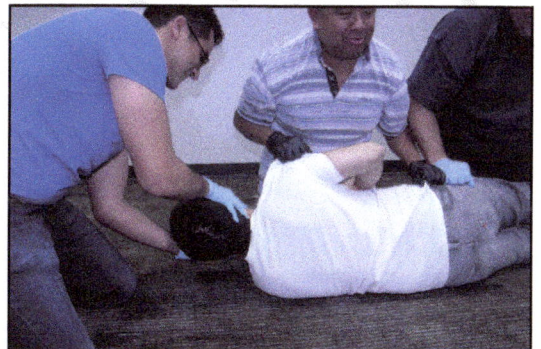

Close up shows victims head in-line with cervical spine.

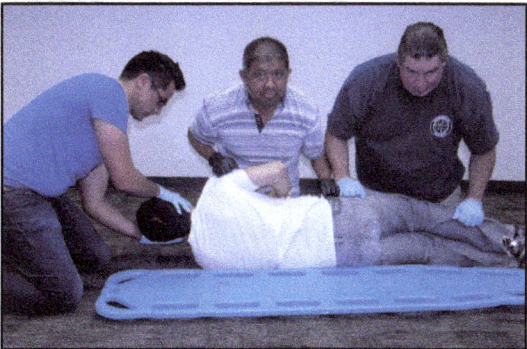

4th Rescuer shows up and places backboard into position. Board is not past the victims head.

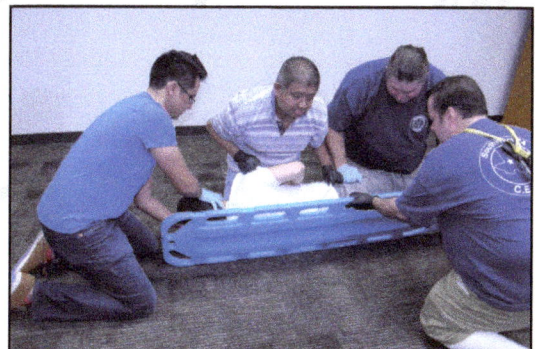

4th Rescuer rolls backboard up to 45º and hold against victim while the 2nd and 3rd rescuer roll victim back onto board. 1st rescuer is still holding c-spine and moving with the victims body as a whole unit.

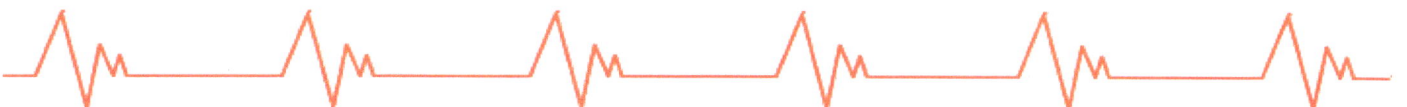

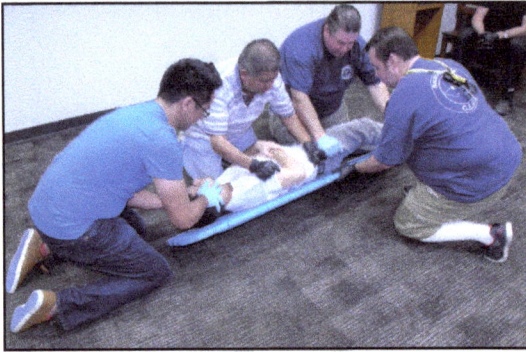

Victim is rolled back to flat position and ready for head-neck to be stabilized.

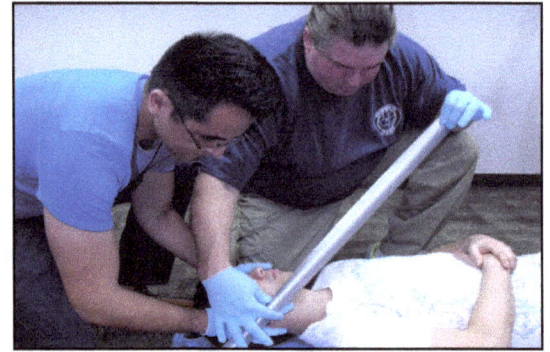

Commercial c-splint are available but during resource shortage always have a roll of duct tape available. Tear off a strip of tape approximately 30" long. Attach one end to the board at a 45º from victim chin area. Pinch tape to fold in-half 4-6" from chin. Let folded tape hold around chin area then fasten tape to other end of backboard.

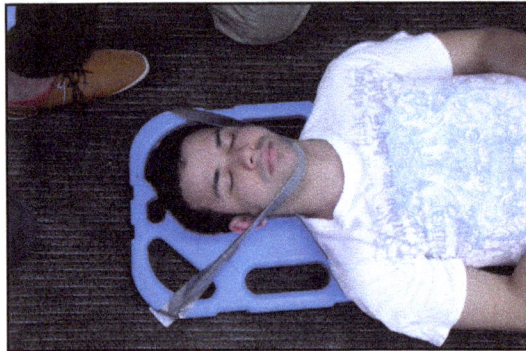

Victims chin is now stabilized and holding in place.

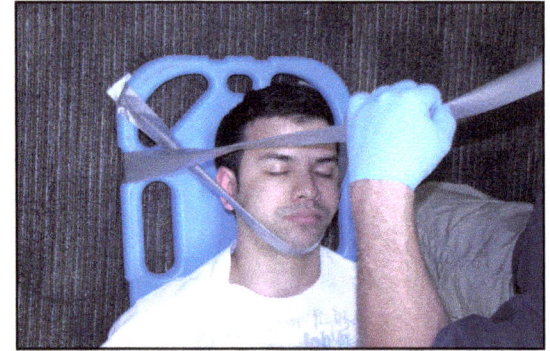

Repeat the same process for the forehead.

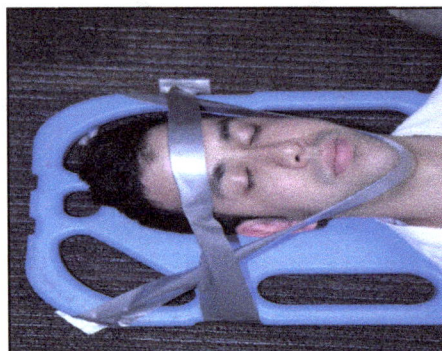

Victim head, neck are now immobilized and can be transported when emergency services arrives.

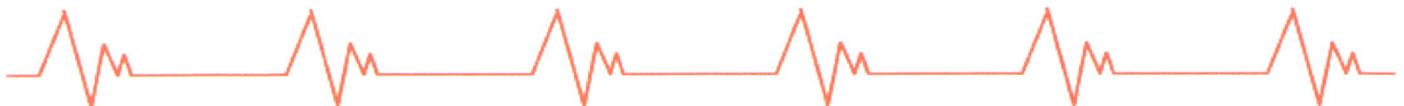

BACK-BOARD LIFT AND CARRY

After most victims are stabilized and immobilized they can be removed from the scene. The following indicates safety steps and guidelines to help the layperson know how to lift, move and carry a victim.

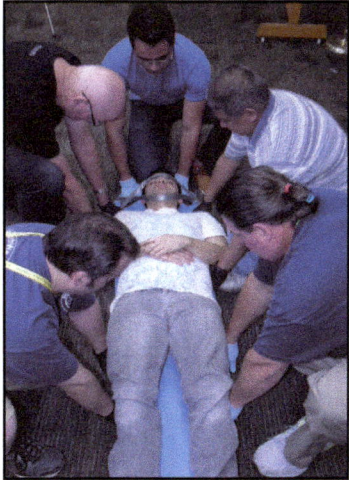

Begin with 5 Rescuers. Size of victim may require 2 additional. Each Rescuer is positioned 2 at head-shoulders. 2 rescuers positioned at knees lower legs area.

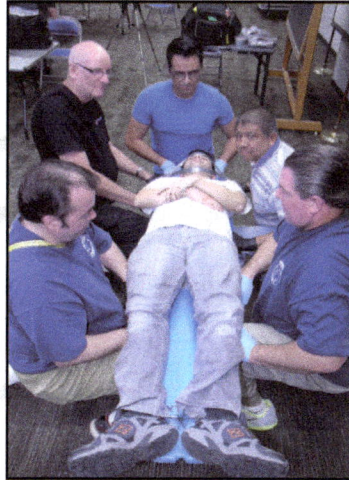

Rescuer 1 gives command. This person is normally at the head of the victim since they can see all rescuers clearly. Rescuer 1 gives count down 3 -2 -1- to lift to knee height only.

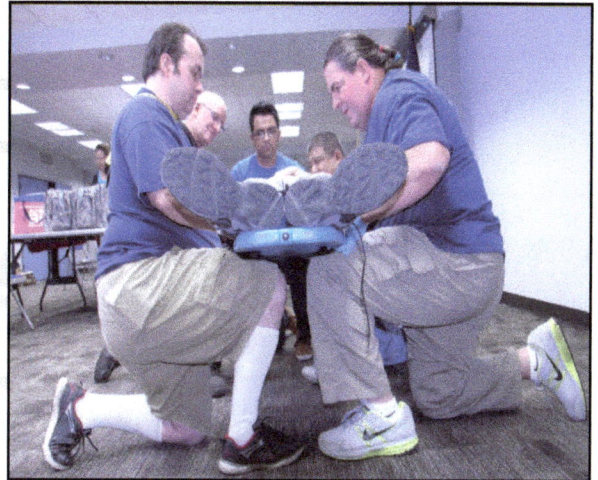

All Rescuers are at knee level and repositioning to complete full lift.

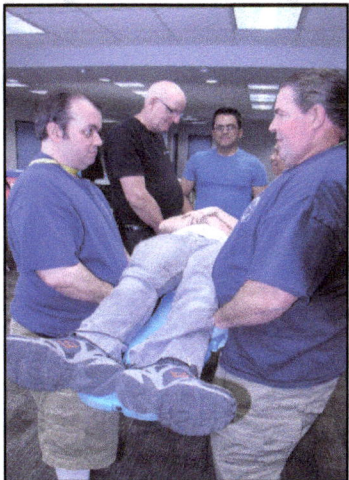

All Rescuers lift completely upward.

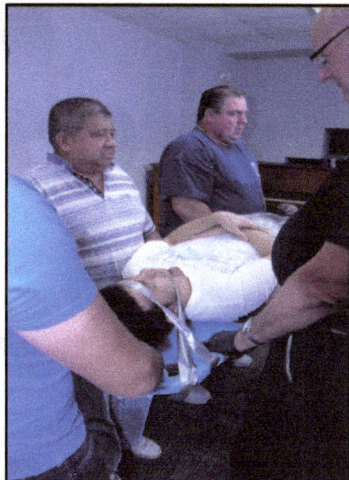

All Rescuers are up and in straight position.

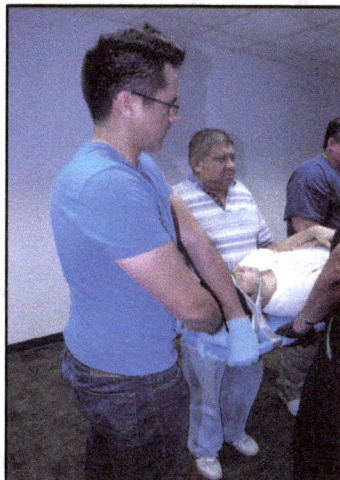

Rescuer 1 at head of victim makes a turn to re-position his heads Hands are now crossing over each other to transport victim.

BACK-BOARD LIFT AND CARRY (P.2)

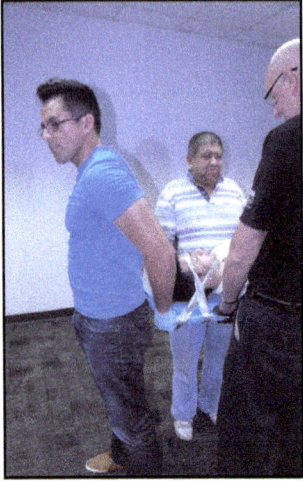

Rescuer 1 turns into position to lead off with transporting victim.

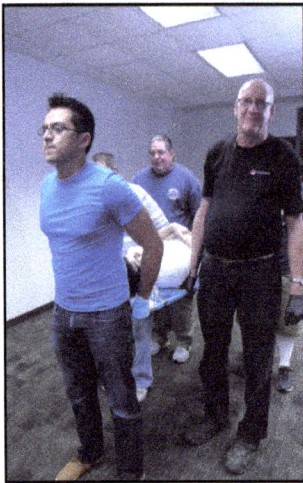

All Rescuers on Right side start off on Right foot. All Rescuers on Left side start victim start off with left foot. This keeps the swaying of the victim off.

Once victim has been transported to a safe location or emergency services area to lower victim back down please remember to reverse these steps.

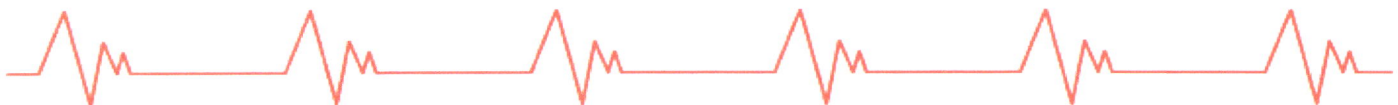

OXYGEN BREATHING OPTIONS

Oxygen is the most critical life support medical assistance a first responder will give. Ensuring proper equipment size, flow and fit are key in successful patient recovery. Adults, Children and Infants require different sizes, shapes and placement adequate flow.

TYPE OF DEVICE	DESCRIPTION	NORMAL FLOW RATE	O2 SATURATIONS	VICTIM LOC
	Normal placement tube ran up and over patients ears loop to nose in upper pull with hose locking under chin area	1 - 5 LPM	24 - 44%	Victims with difficulty breathing Victims claustrophobic about binding face areas
	Pliable, flexible, triangular shape breathing mask that's fits or connects around head covering mouth and nose	5 - 10 LPM	35 - 55%	Victims with difficulty breathing Victims are not breathing Victims in shock
	Oxygen mask with elongated bag with one-way valve between bag and mask. Oxygen is inhaled through bag exhaled air export through one way valve on mask	10 - 15 LPM	70 - 90%	Conscious breathing victims ONLY
	Hand held by Responder self-inflating with one way valve	15 LPM OR HIGHER	80& OR HIGHER	Victim with difficulty breathing Victim who are not breathing Unconscious not breathing

Performing Oxygen on young Children or Infants who are afraid of masks use the "wave" or pass-by" technique. Usually holding the mask about an 1½ to 2" from the face and moving side to side will allow enough oxygen to flow into the mouth or nose to increase oxygen saturation.

Conscious breathing victim can use the BVM, (Bag Valve Mask) for higher concentration of oxygen. You may also squeeze the BVM every other breath less than 10 breaths per minutes. If your victim is rapid breathing, not hyperventilating, squeeze the BVM every second breath to increase oxygen.

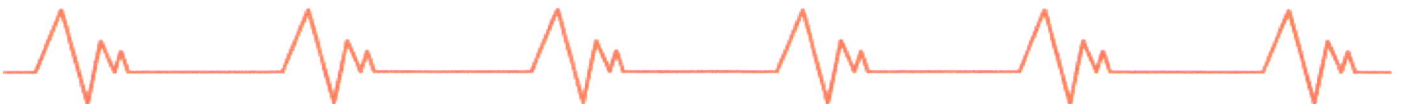

MONITORING OXYGEN SATURATION

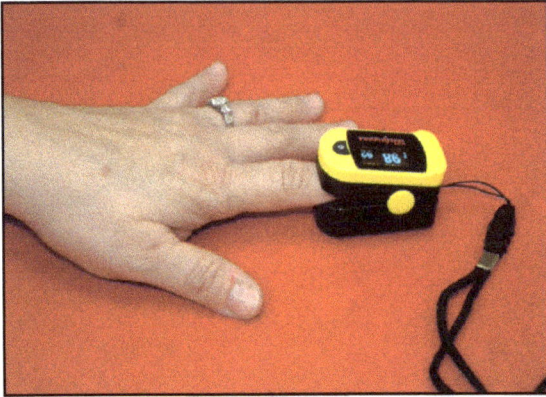

Oximetry, Pulse Oximeters are used to measure the percentage of oxygen the body has in the blood. Normal hemoglobin saturated with oxygen as shown on left, shows the percentage of oxygen (Oximetry reading) recorded using the percentage and the SPO2 (percentage 95-99%)

Pulse Oximetry is an easy valuable tool to speed up the process in evaluating the victim symptoms.

If the victim is complaining of hard breathing, chest pains, shortness of breath and the pulse Oximetry indicates "normal" oxygen reading then add additional oxygen to the victim in every case. Never deny oxygen.

Levels of Oxygen can vary in different climates and altitudes. Be aware of Altitude sickness. If this occurs the fastest treatment is to remove the victim immediately to a lower elevation. Decreasing elevation even by walking down while using oxygen increases volume in capacity.

RANGE	OXYGEN SATURATION	METHOD OF DELIVERY
NORMAL	95 - 100% SPO2	NONE
MILD - NORMAL HYPOXIA	91 - 94% SPO2	NASAL CANNULA OR RESUSCITATION MASK
MODERATE - MILD HYPOXIA	88 - 90% HYPOXIA	NON-REBREATHER MASK OR BVM
SEVERE HYPOXIA	≤ 85% - SPO2	NON-REBREATHER MASK OR BVM

Several "OPTIONS" to use the Oximetry Probe in case of damage or bleeding maybe be earlobe, toes. While monitoring the victim and the pulse indictor and Oximetry read high levels of oxygen you may reduce the oxygen LPM but do not remove the oxygen until EMS arrives.

Obstructions reducing proper readings for Oximetry's:

- Smoking
- Cardiac Arrest
- Movement of motion during evaluation of testing
- Carbon monoxide Poisoning
- Finger nail polish
- Diabetes
- Sickle cell
- Shock

These are a few signs that may interfere with proper reading. In every case if oxygen is available place victim with minimum saturation until EMS arrives.

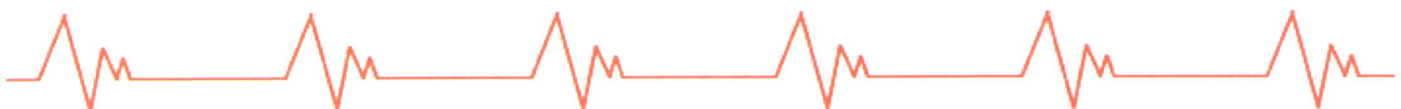

PROPER PLACEMENT OF RESUSITATION MASK OR CHILD

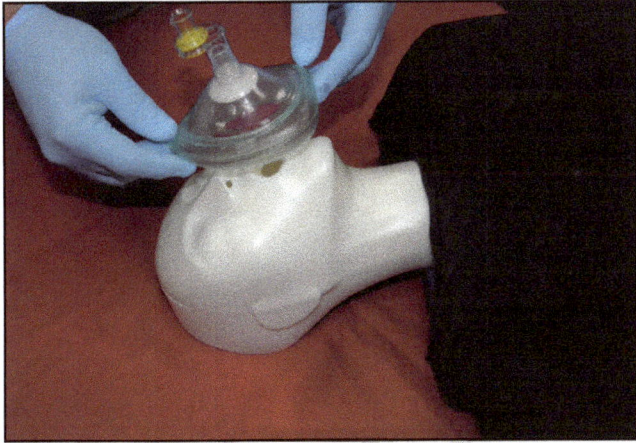

Proper placement of Resuscitation Mask on Adult or Child should fit firmly. Mask should be point towards nose covering nose fitting firmly on face. One-way valve should be rotated so the valve is closest to the rescuer breathing at the forehead of the victim.

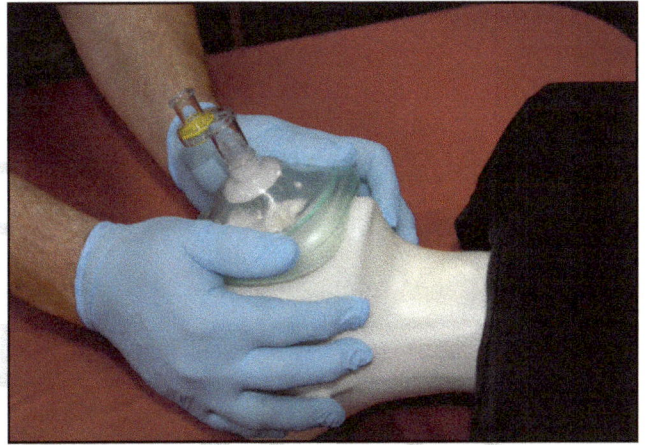

Once mask in in place, use finger tips to hold firmly along lower jaw line and place thumbs firmly on rim on mask to make a tight seal. This prevents air from escaping and allows for maximum oxygen intake.

The rescuer can see the chest rise and fall from this position.

PROPER PLACEMENT OF RESUSITATION MASK INFANT

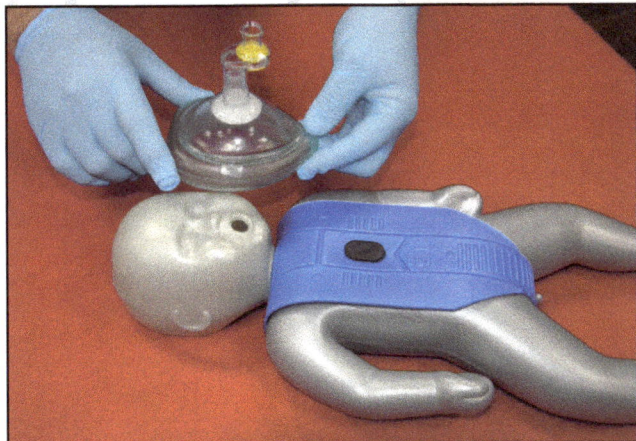

When using Resuscitation mask, one size fits all, completely turn the mask 180% so the point is on the infant's chin. The valve is placed over the Infant's mouth and nose providing direct resuscitation.

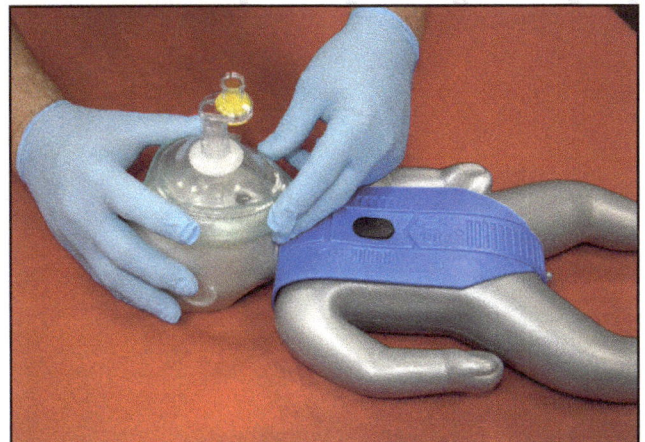

Maintaining a proper open airway with the infants head tilted upward and back at 60% allows for easy air access. Place fingers firmly and lightly around chin line and thumb and index finger along upper jaw line to hold mask in place.

The chest can be seen rising and falling easy from this position.

PREPARING THE OXYGEN CYLINDER

Remove the Cylinder from the case or rack. Handle by throating the bottle on the lower and upper body.

Once you have completely visually inspected the unit 360% check the valve opening for dirt or objects.

Check the cylinder. Look for small particles or debris.

Remove the Valve from the case.

Remove the "O" ring and place in protective zip lock bag until ready to install.

"Quick Turn" the valve for whistle-blow air to clear the piston area.

Attach the "O" ring in place then slide the O2 valve on the neck aligning the air allotted holes. Normally 2 prongs will extend to "catch" in place for proper alignment.

Use only your hands to tighten the O2 valve into place. This will prevent a "pressure lock".

Once cylinder valve is in place open valve slow listening for sounds of air. If you hear sound of air turn off, wait 2 seconds, rehand tighten valve, repeat check.

Turn cylinder over on side to look at valve to check reading on air gauge
.

Some refill stations will always be off by a couple pounds of pressure. It's important to always check your equipment and O2 supply before any event to know your limit on time when supplying O2.

Connect the air-line to the breather mask. Once this is performed then connect the line to the valve on the O2 tank.

Once the plastic tubing has been installed, recheck for kinks or twists in the line.

Replace tank, line and mask back into carrying bag or case.

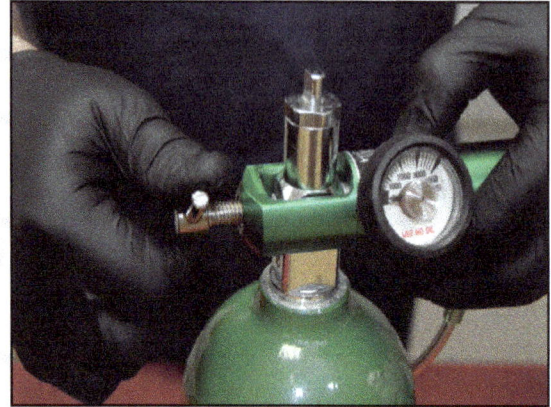

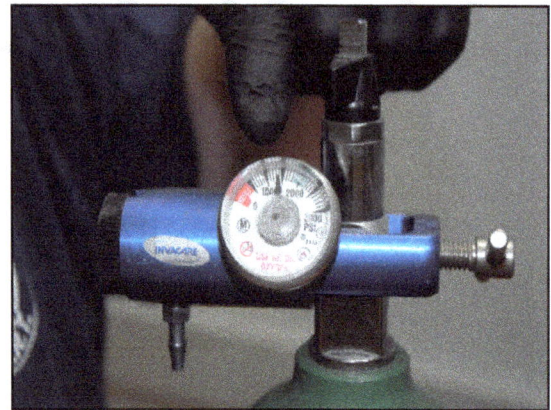

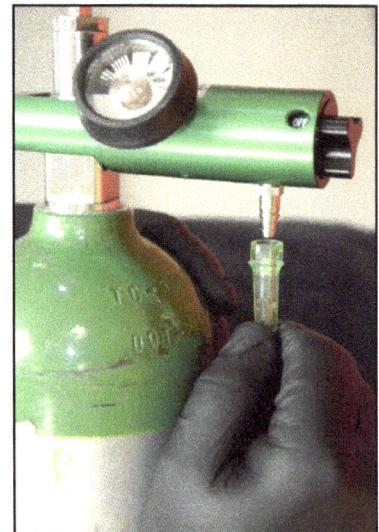

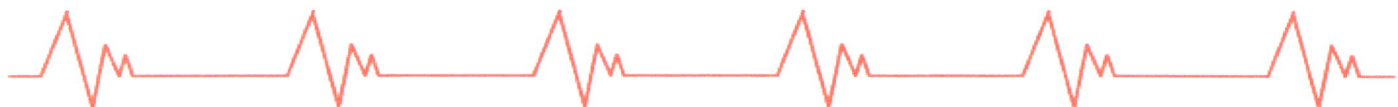

EMERGENCY O2

Each situation and event calls for special circumstances to be made in seconds. When administering O2 normal tanks hold over 2000 PSI. Vendors often get tanks filled above this number. Tanks falling below 180 PSI are consider "used" and should not be used unless on emergency backup.

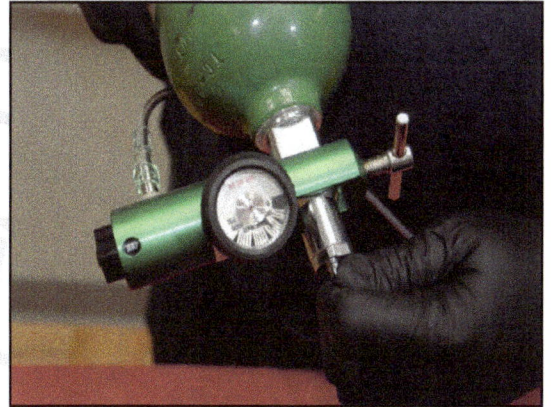

FAST TRACK

In situations where O2 is being applied, remember these FAST Numbers:
1 – 5 – 10 – 15

Flo-Rate

Start with the Nose	1-5 LPM	(Nasal Cannula)
Start with the Mouth	5-10 LPM	(Resuscitation MASK)
Start with the Chin	10-15 LPM	(Non-Rebreather Mask)

If BVM is used start with 15 LPM

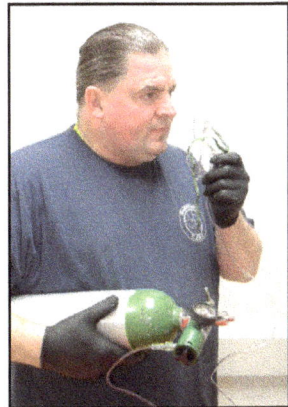

Double check the O2 flow by listening to the flow through

Apply the Mask(s) on the victim. Monitor the victim and watch for signs of panic or shock. Increasing the flow of O2 can decrease panic attacks as with talking to victim keeping them calm.

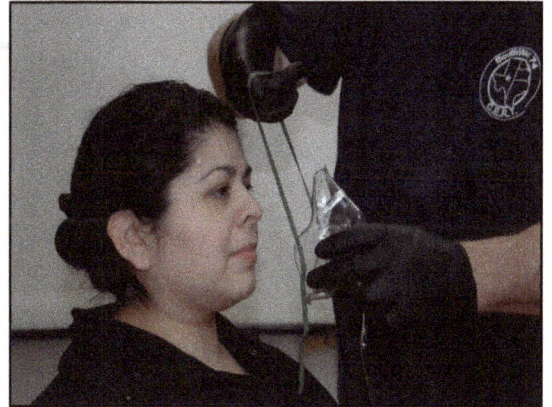

Recheck the Pulse Oximetry levels every 4-5 minutes until EMS arrives. Once you maintain a flow of SPO2 of 98 – 100% you may adjust your flow down to 1 – 5 LPM monitoring your victim LOC and responsiveness.

SAFETY PRECAUTIONS WHEN USING OXYGEN CYLINDERS

- Pressurized tanks have to be checked every 5 years and stamped for verification.

- Check for unusual sounds, leaks, dents, corrosion

- **Never** stand cylinders upright

- **Never** pick up cylinder by valves or hoses

- **Never** place near heat, fires, exhausts

- **Never** grease, oil or lubricate opening, gauges, valves

- **Never** use AED's around flowing Oxygen, Remove from victim before initiating shock

- **Never** remove any tag or check list for inspection on cylinders

INTENTIONALLY LEFT BLANK

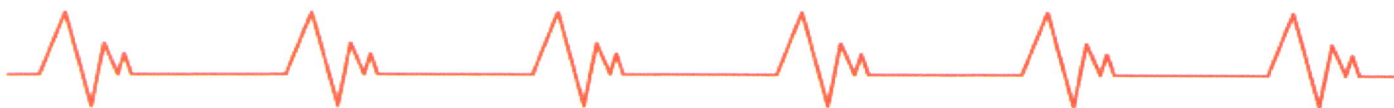

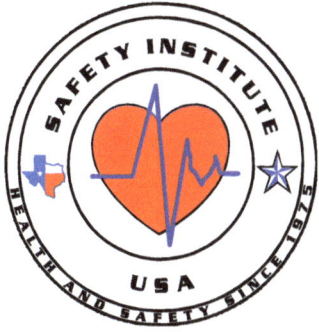

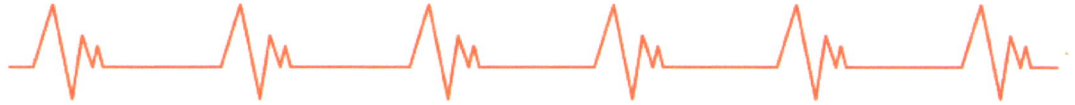

IMPORTANT MESSAGE

This course is for non-professionals only and is not intended for advanced certification. The advanced courses cover more information and in detail. Certificate of "has completed" does not imply future performance or issuance of license. In all emergencies calling EMS/9-1-1 is essential.

EMERGENCY FIRST AID© – BASIC NON-PROFESSIONAL

This is an overview, condensed fact-sheet version of the full-length course! This course is designed to make the rescuer aware of the different types of emergencies. This course due to physical limitation and the American Disabilities Act restricts certain skills from being performed. Remember as a non-license professional your goal is safety first. Always call EMS/9-1-1 in an emergency.

BLEEDING

Definition: Bleeding is the loss of blood from the body. Bleeding may be external or internal.

External Bleeding occurs from open wounds outside the body. Types of open wounds include: abrasions, incisions, lacerations, punctures, avulsion, crushing injuries.

   FIRST AID for this type of bleeding: MOST IMPORTANT – STOP THE BLEEDING, prevent shock, prevent infection (TOURNIQUETS SHOULD NOT BE USED UNLESS DEATH IS IMMINENT).

Internal Bleeding occurs from wounds inside the body. Types of wounds include: small bruises, lung punctures, heart failure, broken blood vessels, fractures bones.

   FIRST AID for this type of bleeding: Apply cold packs to prevent swelling and to slow internal bleeding (DO NOT PUT ICE DIRECTLY ON THE SKIN).

SHOCK

Shock is a condition in which there is loss of effective circulating blood volume. Inadequate organ and tissue perfusion results, ultimately causing cellular metabolic derangements. In all emergency situations, it is wise to anticipate shock before it develops. Any injured person should be assessed immediately to determine the presence of shock.

Common Causes of Shock: bleeding, poisoning, insect bites, snake bites, electrical shock, burns, severe injuries, psychological trauma, heart attack, and other medical conditions.

Signs and Symptoms: pale or bluish lips, gums, and fingernails. Clammy skin in touch, spotted in color. Weakness. Hard to breath or irregular gasps. Can include anxiety, thirst, and nausea.

   FIRST AID for shock: Keep victim lying still but comfortable. Cover them with a blanket to maintain body temperature.

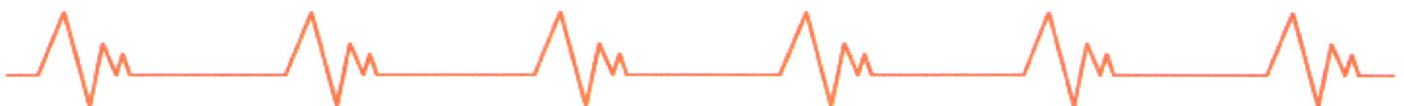

BURNS

First, and foremost, on all burns: Never put ICE on burns. Submerge all burns in cool tap water for fifteen (15) minutes, then wrap with a moist bandage. KEEP BANDAGE MOIST. Never pop a blister. Treat for shock. Call EMS/9-1-1 for severe burns. Never use butter, margarine, or a petroleum product to cover burned area.

NOSE INJURIES

Severe nose bleeds can be frightening to the victim. It is possible that enough blood can be lost to cause shock.

FIRST AID for nose bleeds: Tip victim's head forward, chin to chest, pinch nose at lowest point. Keep victim calm. IMPORTANT: If you suspect a head, neck, or back injury, DO NOT MOVE THE VICTIM. Keep victim still. It might be necessary to treat for shock.

BITES AND STINGS

People are bitten and stung everyday by insects, spiders, snakes, animals, and marine life. Majority of vector/injected bites and sting rarely cause injury. In some cases people have severe reactions, slow breathing, swelling face, arms and legs. "Anaphylaxis Shock" is a life threatening condition that requires immediate medical help.

How to Treat: Bites on children: Wash bitten area thoroughly with soap and water. DO NOT use antiseptic, ointments or other medications. These may cause an allergic reaction. Put a single ice cube on the area to prevent swelling. Document all bite cases.

Insect Bites and Stings: Ants, bees, wasps, spiders, etc.- Use a dull flat surface to gently move upward and downward on stinger area to remove stinger. Do not use tweezers as this may cause further infection.

Spiders: Seek immediate medical help for bites from Black Widow or Brown Recluse or Scorpions. Treat for shock immediately.

FRACTURES, SPRAINS, STRAINS

As a non-professional, treat all fractures, sprains, and strains as broken limbs. Splint if in doubt. With all suspected fractures it is important to get medical help as fast as possible

FIRST AID for Fractures: IMPORTANT – Do not move the fractured area. Simply splint the break exactly as you find it. Use magazines, rolled up newspapers, or soft bound books to roll around the suspected area. Tie articles above and below the area for immobilization. Treat for shock. **Call EMS/9-1-1.**

FIRST AID for Sprain/Strain: Place ice on the area. IMPORTANT – Never place ice directly on the body. Place ice in wet towel or cloth. In case of injury to the feet: leave shoes on: they act as a splint to help keep pressure on the area and to keep injury from swelling. Not all fractures and breaks are noticed with the eyes, please splint even if you suspect a fracture.

POISONING

A poison is any substance; solid, liquid, or gas, that causes injury or death when introduced into the body. There are four (4) main ways a person can be poisoned; by inhaling, absorbing, injecting, and/or swallowing. IN ALL CASES CALL EMS/9-1-1. You must have permission before administering Syrup of Ipecac; NEVER give this to infants (anyone under 18 months of age). NEVER give this without permission from the doctor. Never dilute without permission from a doctor. Keep a sample of any vomit. Keep all containers from the poison. Never induce vomiting if you see blisters. The most common mistake is people calling the information number in an emergency. The emergency number for poisoning is EMS/9-1-1.

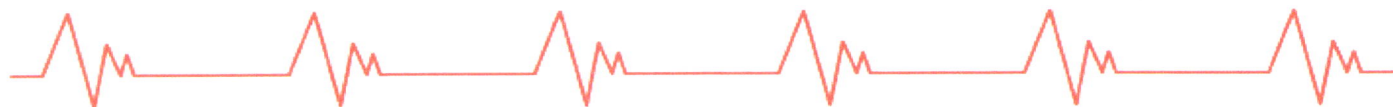

HYPOGLYCEMIA

This is when a person has taken medication but has not eaten. **HYPOGLYCEMIA Signs and Symptoms**: Moist, pale, clammy skin. Profuse cold sweat. May include: hunger, shortness or shallow breathing, confusion, trembling hands, shaking, weakness, dizziness and personality change.

FIRST AID for Hypoglycemia: Give the victim something containing sugar, orange juice, candy, or sugar in any form if they are conscious. This should bring improvements within a few minutes. If this does not bring a change within a few minutes
Call EMS/9-1-1.

SEIZURES

Seizures may be caused by a temporary problem, insulin shock, high fever, viral infection of the brain, head-neck injury, or drug reactions. Epilepsy is usually well controlled with medication, but some people who have it continue to have seizures from time to time. Some individuals have an aura (sensation) before the onset of a seizure. Auras can be sound and vision hallucinations, a strange taste in the mouth, abdominal pain, numbness, or a sense of urgency to move to safety.

Call EMS/9-1-1 if the victim: has multiple seizures, has never had a seizure before, is pregnant, is diabetic, has swallowed a large amount of water, or has a head injury.

In most cases EMS/9-1-1 does not need to be called: if the victim has been diagnosed with seizures, but do the following:

1. Clear the area to prevent further injury; protect the head, use hands under victim's head, let the victim go completely through the seizure(s), NEVER PUT ANYTHING IN THE MOUTH OF THE VICTIM.

2. Open airway after the seizure(s) stop to check A, B, C's, if not breathing begin CPR. Keep the victim calm.

HEATSTROKE

On hot, humid days with no breeze, anyone may be affected by the heat. They may suffer heat stroke, heat exhaustion, or heat cramps. The body temperature can rise so high that brain damage and death may result if the body is not quickly cooled down. Quickly cool the victim's body. Heat stroke requires medical attention.

Signs and Symptoms of Heatstroke: Hot, red skin, very small pupils, and very high body temperature sometimes as high as 105º degrees. Rapid pulse. Confusion or disorientation. Unconsciousness. (Hot, red raise the head)

FIRST AID for heatstroke: Call EMS/9-1-1. Get the person out of the heat and into a cooler place. Immerse him or her in a cool bath, wrap wet sheets around the body and fan it. Reduce temperature to 101º degrees. Give nothing by mouth. Do not give medications.

HEAT EXHAUSTION

Heat Exhaustion is less dangerous than heat stroke. Fluid loss causes blood flow to decrease in the vital organs, resulting in a form of shock. With heat exhaustion, sweat does not evaporate as it should, possibly because of high humidity or too many layers of clothing. As a result, the body is not cooled effectively. (Cool, pale raise the tail)

Signs and Symptoms of Heat Exhaustion: Cool, pale, and moist skin – heavy sweating, dilated pupils, headache, nausea, dizziness, and vomiting. Body temperature will be nearly normal.

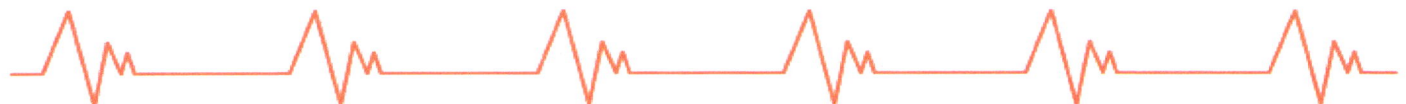

FIRST AID for Heat Exhaustion: Get the person out of the heat. Place him or her in the shock position, remove or loosen the victim's clothing. Cool him or her by fanning and applying cold packs. Use wet towels or sheets. Give the victim ½ glassful of water to drink every 15 minutes, if he or she is fully conscious. These steps should bring improvement within a half hour.

SNAKEBITES

Venomous snakes cause some 8,000 of the 45,000 snakebites that occur each year in the USA and 9 to 15 deaths per year are attributed to these snakebites. Children between the ages of 1 and 9 years are the most likely victims. The greatest number of bites occurs during daylight hours in summer months. Venomous snakebites are medical emergencies. Call EMS/9-1-1.

Signs and Symptoms of Snake bites: Pain mild to moderate. Swelling, discolored skin, dizziness, nausea, drowsiness, sweating, headaches, drooling, thirst, weakness, severe slurred speech, blurred vision, vomiting, convulsions, difficulty breathing.

FIRST AID for Snake bites: Keep the victim calm. Remove all constrictive items such as rings. Keep victim warm. Keep the bitten area below the level of the heart. Apply a clean bandage on the area to minimize the contamination any further. Do NOT place ice or a tourniquet on the area. This may speed up the poison by causing shock. Monitor the victim's C, A, B's. Get help immediately. If you can identify the snake poisonous / non-poisonous advise EMS/9-1-1 or the hospital of its type for antivenin purposes.

FIRE DRILLS

When there is no present danger, follow local routines as prescribed at your location. IMPORTANT: If EMS/911 has been called clear the area immediately to allow easy access. In case of fire-drill make sure everyone knows how and where to go during the drill. IMPORTANT: Never separate the school or business. Have everyone meet at one local point so that a single head count can be presented. This will also tell you if anyone is missing. It is your responsibility to inform all participants of each planned drill and how to proceed.

FOR MORE INFORMATION ON FIRST AID CLASSES OR CPR CLASSES

EMAIL: CLASSES@SAFETYINSTITUTEUSA.ORG

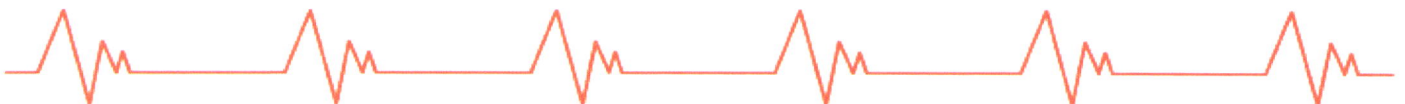

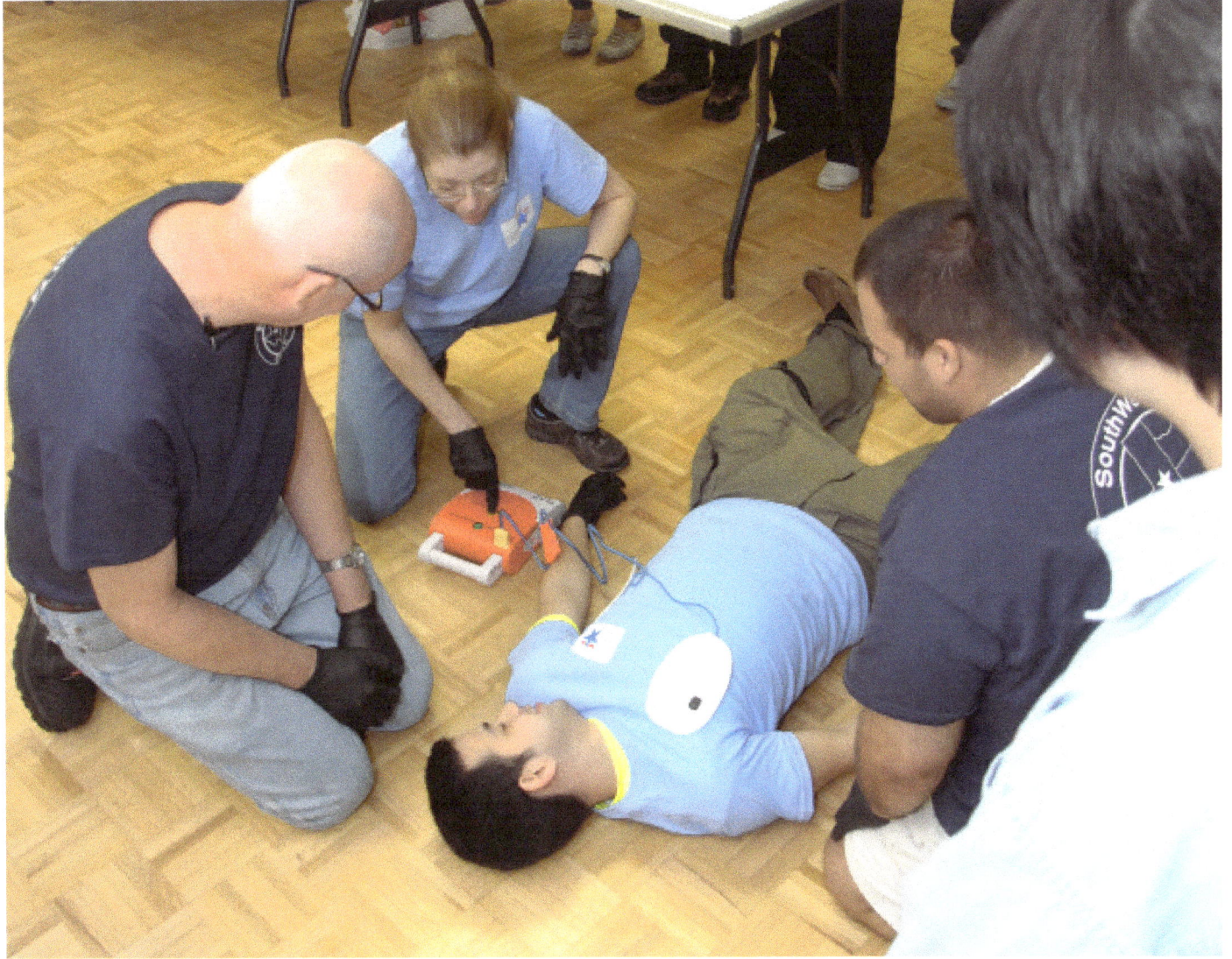

"AED INSTRUCTION"
PHOTOGRAPHER: DAN SLOAN

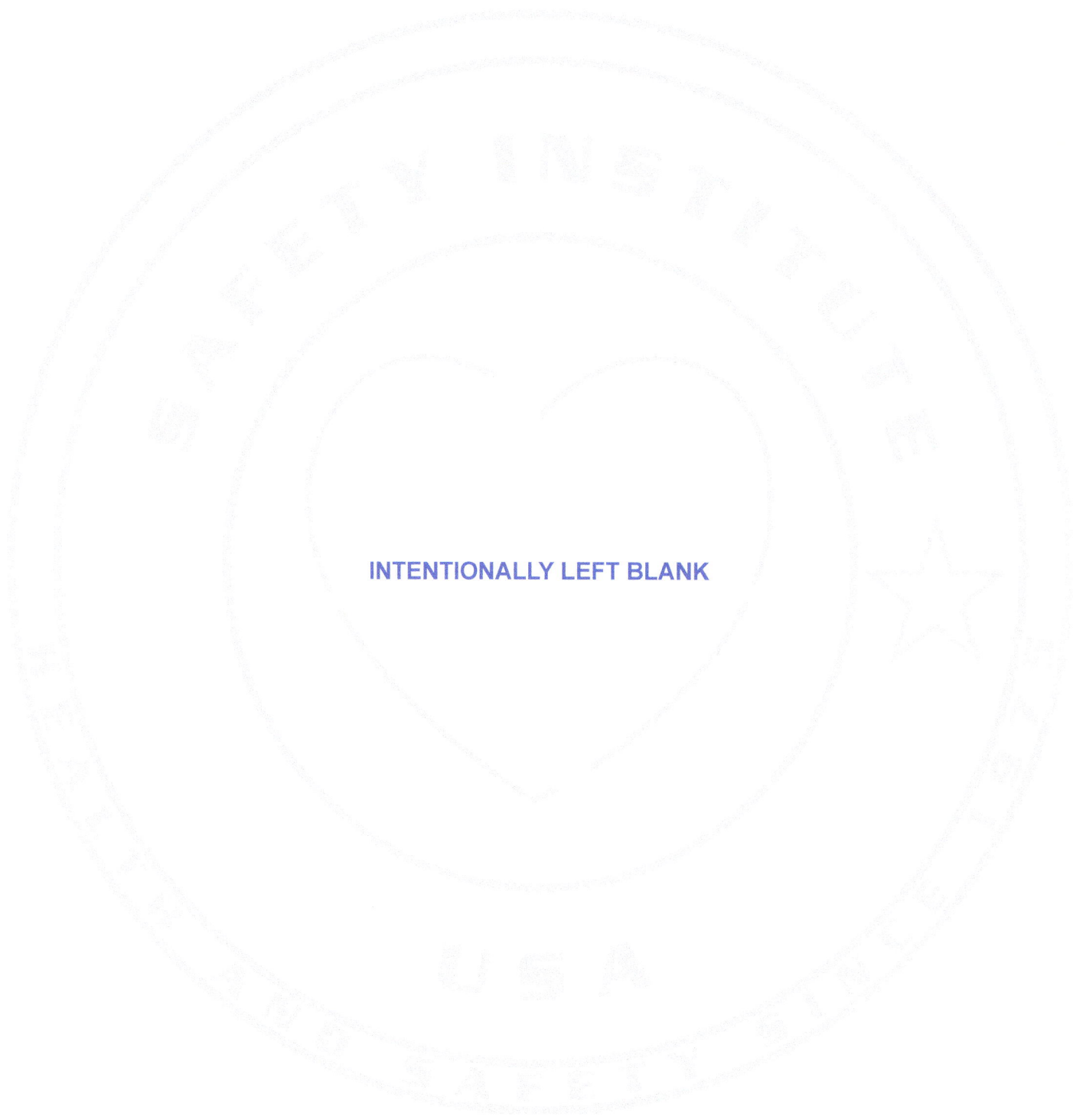

INTENTIONALLY LEFT BLANK

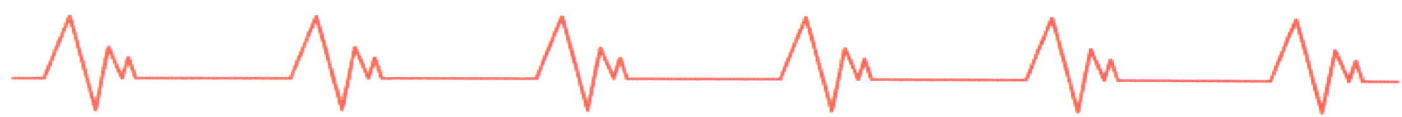

FACTS TO CONSIDER ABOUT CPR

A person who needs CPR will most likely be resuscitated by someone they don't know.

For an ADULT or CHILD, CALL 9 – 1 – 1 before starting CPR

For an INFANT, START CPR immediately, perform CPR for about 2-minutes, then CALL 9 – 1 – 1.

Continue to help the victim until:

- Another trained rescuer takes over from you

- EMS arrives on the scene and takes over from you

- The victim starts breathing on his / her own

If you can't continue CPR because you are tired or hurt

- Roll the victim onto their side into the recovery position

- Keep the victim's airway open

- Resume CPR as able

It is important to give help until EMS arrives.

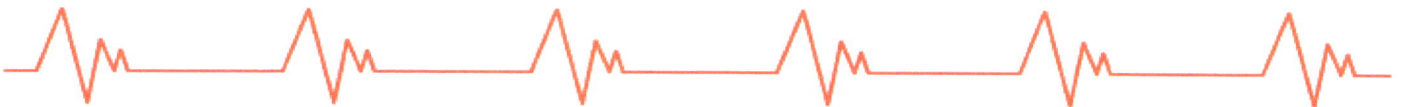

CPR CARDIAC EMERGENCIES

C

In the United States Cardiac Emergencies are high risks. Heart Attacks and cardiac arrest are major causes of death. Learning CPR and providing it in the first few seconds or minutes to someone experiencing a heart problem can be life altering.

P

Recognizing the signs and symptoms of heart problems, Calling 9 – 1 – 1 EMS immediately, and learning how to use the AED, Automated External Defibrillator, are ways to help the victim or injured.

R

Remember that Cardiac arrest happens in Children and Infants as well Adults.

CPR STANDS FOR CARDIO-PULMONARY-RESUSCITATION

KNOWING WHAT TO LOOK FOR OR RECOGNIZING

Leading signs of heart problems are Chest Pain, Pressure in the chest, Discomfort or anxiety, Dizziness, Indigestion, Blurred vision, tingling in hands and arms, and shortness of breath

NOTICING THE OTHER INDICATORS

Men and Women while having the same signs show indications at different ages in life. Women can start as early in the 30's while Men start to show in late 40's early 50's. Women pass off the signs of trouble breathing or sleeping, feeling scared or nervous, new or worse headaches and pain in the belly above the belly button are just a few differences

OTHER INDICATORS

Women are more commonly misdiagnosed when visiting their doctor. Since 2011, doctors have been more aware of the signs of cardiac problems in women

WOMEN TEND TO BE MORE HEALTHY AND CONCERNED OVER THEIR HEALTH THAN MEN.

Having unexplained fatigue, face, jaw or back pains are unusual, but sometimes over-looked even when noticed.

LEARNING WHEN TO CALL EMS 9 - 1 – 1 SHOULD BE CALLED IMMEDIATELY.

Minutes are critical to life saving. Most cardiac victims ignore the onset of the signs and usually die within 2-3 hours for not seeking immediate help.

EARLY DETECTIONS, GIVING MEDICATIONS CAN HELP UNTIL EMS ARRIVES

Victims may have prescribed medications they have not taken, nitroglycerin pills, and irregular heart beat medicines.

DOING THE FOLLOWING

Have the victim rest or stop activity immediately. Loosen clothing.

GIVE ASPIRIN TO HELP EASE THE HEART ATTACK.

If victim is conscious, ask if they are allergic to aspirin. If available give 1 adult aspirin or 2 baby aspirin and monitor victim until EMS arrives.

EARLY DETECTION AND EARLY ACCESS TO EMS IS VITAL.

Beginning CPR quickly can help blood maintain oxygen to the brain. Without proper oxygen brain damage may start to occur within 4 – 6 minutes

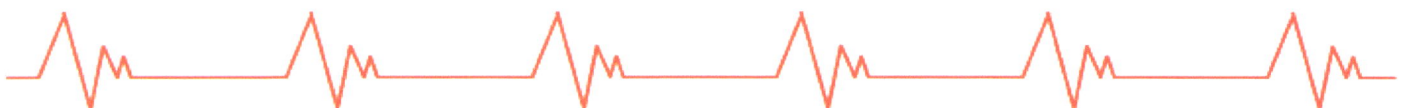

HEART ATTACK

COMMON SIGNS

Chest pain or discomfort. Pains lasting longer than 3-5 minutes then reoccurring. Indigestion and chest pains are similar. Other signs and symptoms of a heart problem:

- Tightness in the chest - one side or the other – or alternating
- Pains in chest like a direct blow or hit
- Muscle spasms in upper chest
- Pain in shoulders, arms, neck, back or stomach.
- Difficulty breathing, shortness of breath, or hard breathing
- Skin color - lighter, gray or light bluish tint

Men vs. Women

Until recently, signs of heart attack in women were often missed. Doctors considered other medical issues were causing women to have signs of indigestion and chest pains. With reevaluation, women are urged to start checking for heart attacks as early as age 35 and men at age 40.

HEART ATTACK SIGNS IN WOMEN

1. Uncomfortable pressure, squeezing, fullness or pain in the center of your chest. It lasts more than a few minutes, or goes away and comes back.
2. Pain or discomfort in one or both arms, the back, neck, jaw or stomach.
3. Shortness of breath with or without chest discomfort.
4. Other signs such as breaking out in a cold sweat, nausea or lightheadedness.
5. As with men, the most common symptom of heart attack in women is chest pain or discomfort. Women are somewhat more likely than men to experience some of the other common symptoms, particularly shortness of breath, nausea/vomiting and back or jaw pain.

If you have any of these signs, don't wait more than five minutes before calling for help.
Call 9-1-1 and get to a hospital right away.

LINKS TO SURVIVAL

Someone experiencing a heart problem is much more likely to survive if:
- CALL 9 – 1 – 1 as soon as you recognize a Heart attack or Stroke
- PERFORM CPR if necessary to provide oxygen to the brain and organs.
- USE an AED to Defibrillate or re-start the heartbeat.
- TREATMENT by Emergency care at the closest hospital or ambulance to treatment is critically important

QUICK CHECK

Once you notice a victim in distress, begin evaluating immediately.
- Call 9-1-1 immediately.
- CHECK the area – is it safe for you to approach the victim?

START EMERGENCY RESCUE STEPS IMMEDIATELY.
- LOOK for bleeding. - - STOP any BLEEDING as QUICKLY as possible
- LOOK for signs of breathing - - START CPR .. Perform CPR and Rescue Breathing

These steps are critical. Think of it as if it were your car. If you have a tank full of gas but you have an oil leak, no matter how much gas you have without oil your engine will never run
.
CPR is a combination of skills taught. If the heart stops, providing combination of chest compressions and breaths are essential to proving oxygen and circulation for the body. Early AED is critical to help boost the survival rate in victims. Indications have shown that CPR alone is not enough. Proving early and fast defibrillation, AED, can increase the chances of survival. Also, when trying to assist, it is important to follow some safety guidelines.

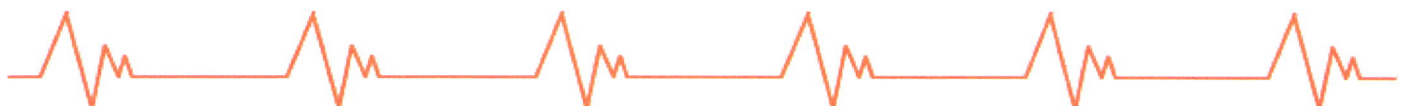

STROKE

A stroke happens about every 40 seconds. Each year, about 795,000 Americans have a stroke. Do you know the warning signs?

If you do have stroke warning signs, this means your brain isn't getting the blood it needs. Damage may be temporary or permanent. For example, you might lose the ability to speak, but recover it with time. You might have partial or complete weakness, for example, in the use of an arm or leg.

The important thing is what you do if stroke symptoms happen. The sooner the treatment, the less chance of serious damage to the brain. And this means less chance of permanent disability.

COMMON SIGNS

Sometimes symptoms of stroke develop gradually. But if you are having a stroke, you are more likely to have one or more sudden warning signs like these:

- Numbness or weakness in your face, arm, or leg, especially on one side
- Confusion or trouble understanding other people
- Trouble speaking
- Trouble seeing with one or both eyes
- Trouble walking or staying balanced or coordinated
- Dizziness
- Severe headache that comes on for no known reason

TYPES OF STROKES

Stroke symptoms may differ, depending upon the type of stroke, where it occurs in the brain, and how severe it is. A less severe stroke may be more difficult to recognize

An ischemic stroke happens when a vessel supplying blood to the brain becomes blocked. It can happen for a variety of reasons. For example, fatty deposits in arteries (atherosclerosis) can cause blood clots to form. Sometimes a blood clot forms in the heart from an irregular heartbeat called atrial fibrillation. It then travels to a place where it blocks an artery supplying the brain.

A hemorrhagic stroke happens when a weakened blood vessel ruptures and bleeds into the brain. This can also happen for a variety of reasons.

A transient ischemic attack (TIA) is a "mini stroke" from a temporary blockage. Although a TIA doesn't cause permanent brain damage, it may cause stroke warning signs, which may last minutes or even hours. Think of this as a warning sign you shouldn't ignore.

WHAT TO DO IF YOU HAVE SYMPTOMS OF STROKE

Remember that a stroke is a medical emergency. Sometimes it is even called a brain attack.

- Don't ignore stroke warning signs – even if you have just one warning sign or if symptoms are mild or go away.
- Don't wait! Every minute counts.
- Call 911 or emergency medical services (EMS) if you have one or more symptoms for more than a few minutes. An ambulance can get you to a hospital without delay.
- Check the time when symptoms begin. This is important information to share when you arrive at the hospital.

What if you're with someone else who might be having stroke symptoms but you're not sure?

TAKE CHARGE AND CALL 911.

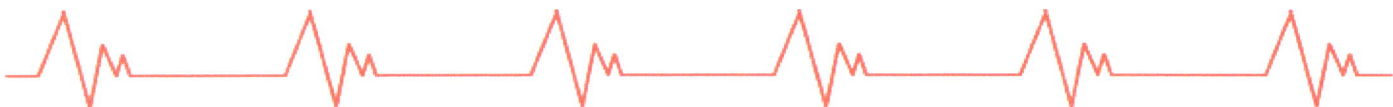

	CDC CENTERS FOR DISEASE CONTROL, ATLANTA GEORGIA 2013
	PROPER DISINFECTING MANIKINS BEFORE EACH USE IN CLASSROOM SETTING
	(The following recommendations for decontaminating manikins use in CPR training were furnished to the Emergency Medical Services Program by the United States Center for Disease Control, Atlanta, Georgia)
1.	The manufacturer's recommendations and provision for sanitary practices should be thoroughly examined.
2.	Students should be told in advance that the training sessions will involve "close physical contact" with their fellow students.
3.	Students should not actively participate in training sessions if they have dermatologic lesions on the hands or in oral or circumoral areas; are known to be hepatitis B carriers; have upper-respiratory-traction infections or AIDS (or evidence of HTLV III/LAV infection); or the student has reason to believe that he or she has been exposed to or is in the active stage of any infectious process.
4.	If more than one CPR manikin is used in class, students should be assigned in pairs, with each pair having contact with only one manikin. This limits exposure. A one-to-One manikin is ideal for prevention.
5.	All persons responsible for CPR training should be thoroughly familiar with hygienic concepts, as well as the procedures for cleaning and maintaining manikins and accessories. Manikins should be inspected routinely for signs of physical deterioration, such as cracks or tears in plastic surfaces, which prevent thorough cleaning. Manikins clothes, hair should be washed periodically or whenever visibly soiled.
6.	In order to limit the potential for disease transmission during the professional rescuer "switching procedure" the second student taking over ventilation should simulate it instead of blowing onto the manikin.
7.	When practicing the "obstructed airway procedure" the finger sweep should either be simulated or done on a manikin whose airway was decontaminated before the procedure will be decontaminated afterwards.
8.	Each time a different student uses the manikins, the individual protective shield, face guard if used should be changed or decontaminated. After a potentially contaminating procedure, the manikins face and inside mouth should be wiped clean vigorously with clean absorbent material (e.g.4"x4" gauze pad) wetted with a solution of chloride bleach ¼ cup to gallon on water. Persons allergic to bleach may use alcohol wipes as necessary. The surface should remain wet for a period of 30 seconds before they are wiped dry and a second piece of absorbent placed on the area. Although highly bactericidal, alcohol are not broad spectrum agents; their use here is recommended primarily as an aid in mechanical cleaning and because some persons for the odor or hypochlorite objectionable. Little viable microbial contamination is likely after the cleaning procedure.
9.	At the end of the class, the procedures listed below should be followed to avoid drying of contamination on manikin surfaces. • Disassembled the manikin as directed by manufacture • As indicated, thoroughly wash all external surfaces (also reusable protective face shield with warm soapy water and brushes. • Rinse all surfaces with fresh water. • Wet all surfaces with a sodium hypochlorite solution having at least 500 ppm free available chlorite (1/4 cup) liquid house hold bleach (approximately 5% sodium hypochlorite) per half gallon of tap water. This solution must be made fresh daily) This solution must be made fresh every day before class. • Rinse with fresh water and immediately dry all dry all external and internal surfaces.
10.	Persons responsible for the use and maintenance should not totally rely of disinfectants for protection from cross-infection. Microbial contamination is easily removed from smooth, nonporous surfaces by using disposable cleaning cloths moistened with a detergent solution. There is no evidence that a soaking procedure alone in any liquid is as effective as the same procedure accompanied by vigorous scrubbing.
11.	If manikins and participants ratios allow preferably a one-to-one manikins is the easiest way to prevent cross contamination.
12.	Use isopropyl alcohol a secondary backup to allergic reactions to bleach cleaning.

3 POSITIONS OFTEN USED FOR RESCUE BREATHING

3 types of rescue breathing are; mouth - to – mouth, mouth - to- nose, mouth - to – stoma. All are acceptable rescue breathing styles. Situations may arise where these will me necessary to perform rescue breathing.

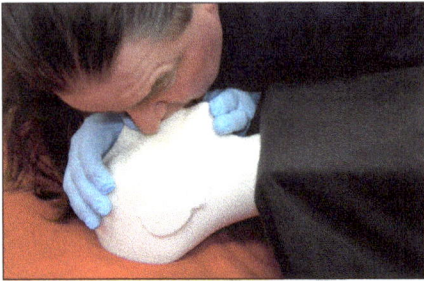

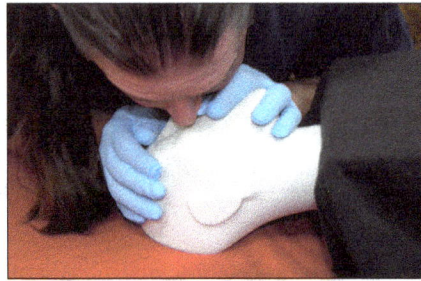

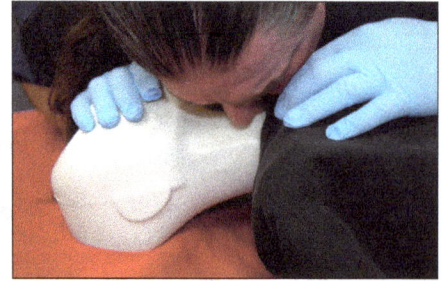

| MOUTH - TO - MOUTH | MOUTH - TO - NOSE | MOUTH - TO - STOMA |

COMPRESSIONS ONLY CPR – HANDS ONLY – NO BREATHS

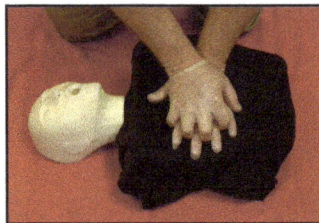

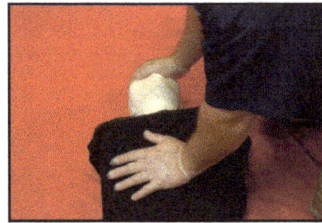

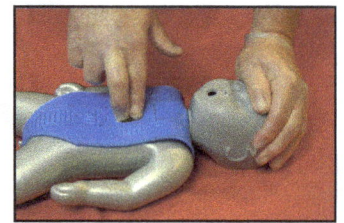

CPR	ADULT	CHILD	INFANT
HAND PLACEMENT	2 hands in center of chest, mid-to-lower sternum	1 hand in center of chest, mid-to-lower sternum	2-3 fingers in center of chest below nipple line
COMMPRESSION DURATION	30 compressions – 20-25 seconds, 5 sets	30 compressions – 20-25 seconds, 5 sets	30 compressions – 20-25 seconds, 5 sets
COMPRESSION DEPTH	2 inches (1½-2") (2 hands)	1 inch (1-1 ½") (I hand)	½" (½ - 1") (2-3 fingers)
RECHECK	5 SETS	5 SETS	5 SETS

Many Reasons why lay rescuers will not want to breathe on the victim are: strangers, blood on the face, scared, or afraid to name a few.

Compressions ratios and depths are vital to supporting enough oxygen and blood circulation in the body until medical helps arrives.

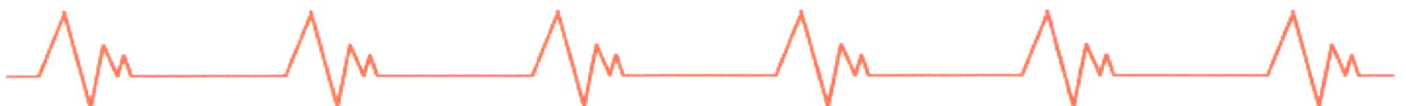

CPR - 6 STEPS FOR ADULTS

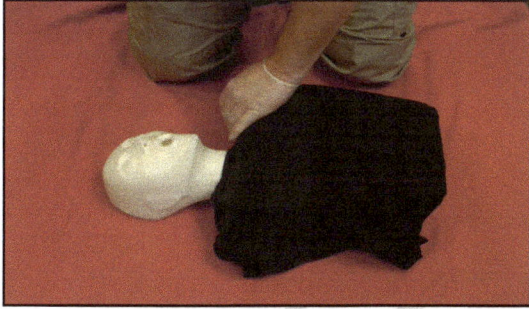

Shake shoulders firmly, "loudly, ask victim, "Are you okay?"

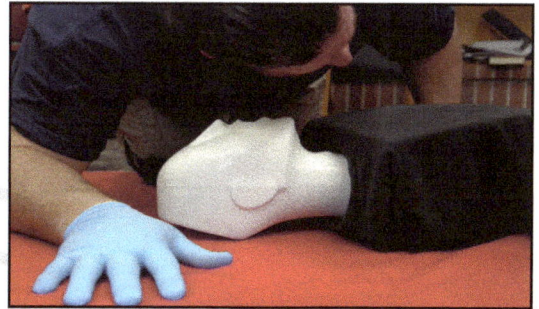

"Quick" Check for Breathing, Look, Listening and Feeling for Breaths. Do Not touch the victim at this point.

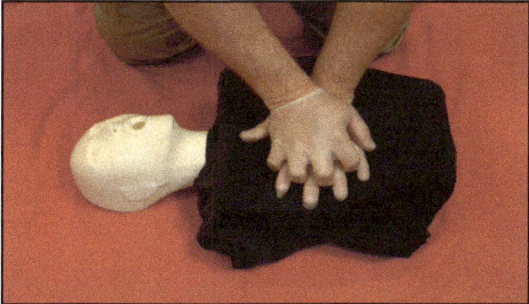

If not Breathing IMMEDIATELY begin CPR, Begin 30 Chest compressions. Place the heel on one hand down in center of chest. Then, place the other hand on top of the first hand. Use "Both hands to compress". (Notice one knee is in-line with victim's ear and other knee is in-line with hands on chest.) Compress 1 - 1½ inches. (100 compressions per minute is the optimal goal.)

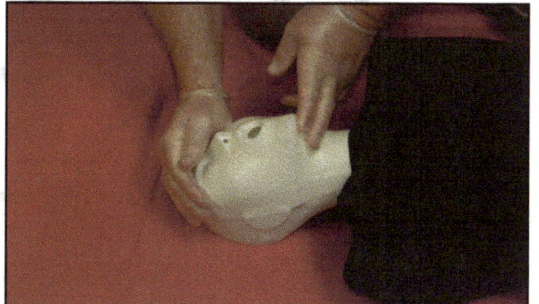

Open the "Air-Way", using Head-Chin-lift method. Never touch the neck.

Place 1 hand on the forehead and 2 fingers under the boney part of the chin. Tilt chin upward and back.

Mouth should be angled back at a slight pitch to allow easy breathing.

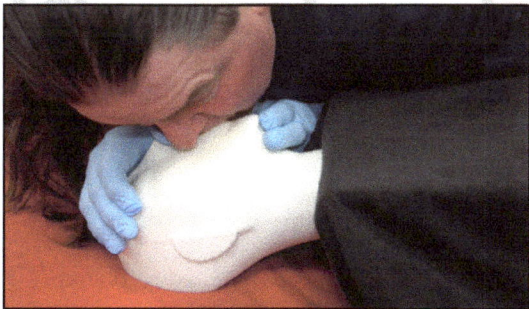

Check Breathing for 5 seconds. If not breathing give 2 breaths, followed immediately with 30 chest compressions performing 5 sets of 30 compressions and 2 breaths.

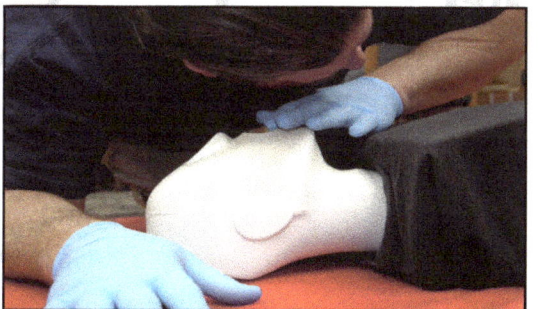

Recheck victim for breathing for 5 seconds. If not breathing continue CPR. "If you determine breaths" keep airway open and monitor victim every 2 minutes for reassessment until medical help arrives.

CHOKING CONSCIOUS / UNCONSCIOUS RESCUE SKILLS FOR THE ADULT

In all Choking Emergency situations getting Oxygen to the brain is critically important. Without oxygen the brain within 4 - 6 minutes is in danger of brain damage is possible. Within 6 – 8 minutes brain damage is likely. Over 10 minutes irreversible brain damage is certain.

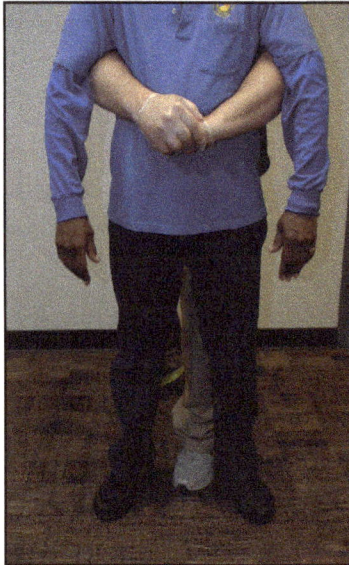

Conscious Choking

Position your feet to stabilize the victim. Rescuer's ankle should be between the victim ankles feet. Rescuer's rear foot should be back enough to brace rescuer and victim.

When placing hands around victims waist just at the belt line, cup the other hand over the inner hand. Inner hand is rolled inward, thumb laid across index finger, not tucked in.
Squeeze inward and upward 5 times.

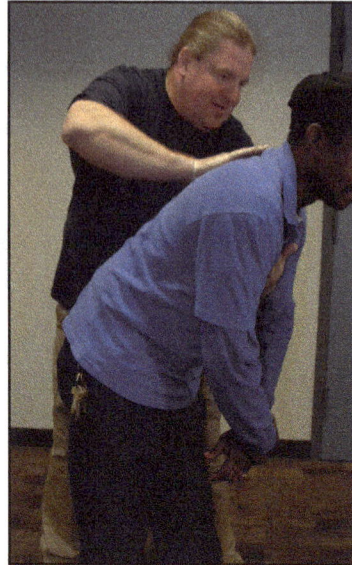

Continue with 5 back blows leaning the victim forward, positioning the head and shoulders lower to expel the object.
One hand should be placed in the victim's upper chest to support the victim.

Using the other hand, heel of the palm continue with 5 blows between the shoulder blades.

If Victims becomes Unconscious start with "Opening the Airway" then "Looking" and "Sweeping the Airway" every time on the Adult/Child.

IF VICTIM BECOMES UNCONSCIOUS

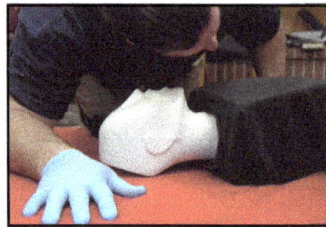

Open, Airway, Use "Index-Pointer finger" to insert into the unconscious victims mouth on side away from you then sweep back in a hooking motion.

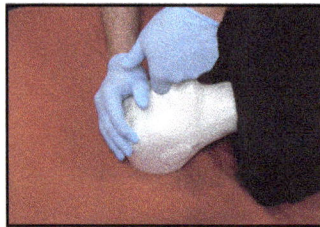

After sweeping the mouth and you see no object or no object was removed begin:

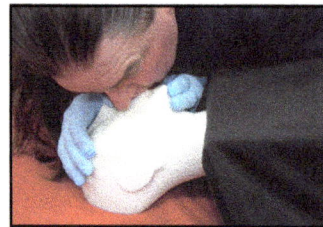

Try and Give 2 breaths. If air did not go in immediately starts chest compressions.

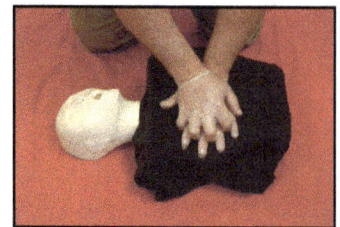

Places your hands on the chest and compress the chest 30 times.

REPEAT the Steps. "Open, Sweep, Breath, Compressions until object comes out or emergency medical help arrives. If victims starts breathing, leave in Shock Position and monitor.

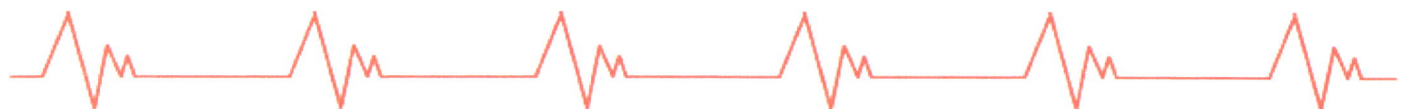

CPR - 6 STEPS FOR THE CHILD

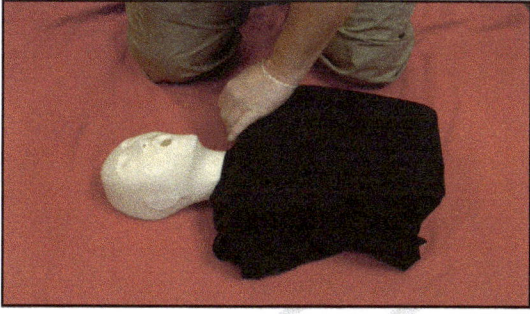

Shake shoulders firmly, "loudly, ask victim, "Are you okay?"

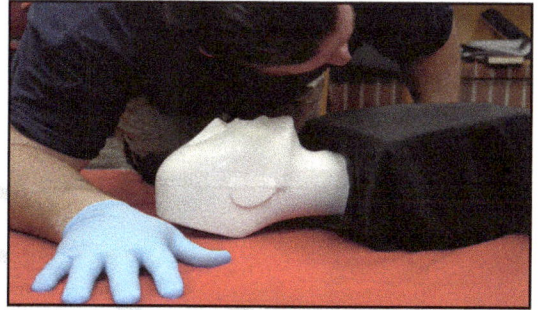

"Quick" Check for Breathing, Look, Listening and Feeling for Breaths. Do Not touch the victim at this point.

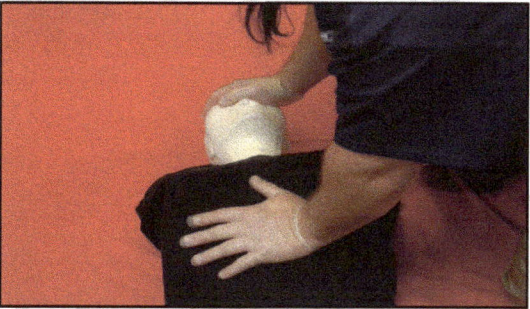

If not Breathing IMMEDIATELY begin CPR, Begin 30 Chest compressions. Place the heel on one hand down in center of chest. Then, place the other hand on top of the first hand. Use "Both hands to compress". (Notice one knee is in-line with victim's ear and other knee is in-line with hands on chest.) Compress 1 - 1½ inches. (100 compressions per minute is the optimal goal.)

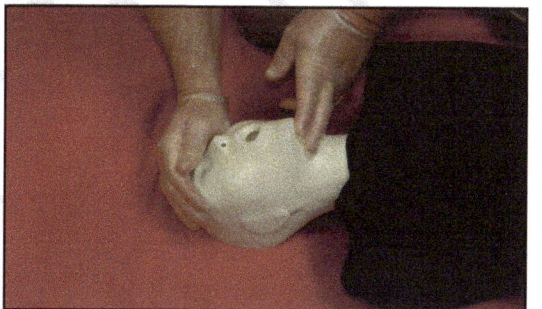

Open the "Air-Way", using Head-Chin-lift method. Never touch the neck.

Place 1 hand on the forehead and 2 fingers under the boney part of the chin. Tilt chin upward and back.

Mouth should be angled back at a slight pitch to allow easy breathing.

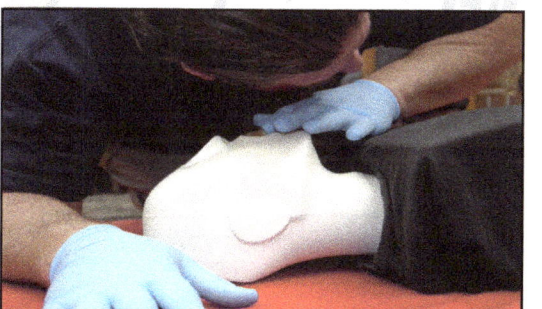

Check Breathing for 5 seconds. If not breathing give 2 breaths, followed immediately with 30 chest compressions performing 5 sets of 30 compressions and 2 breaths.

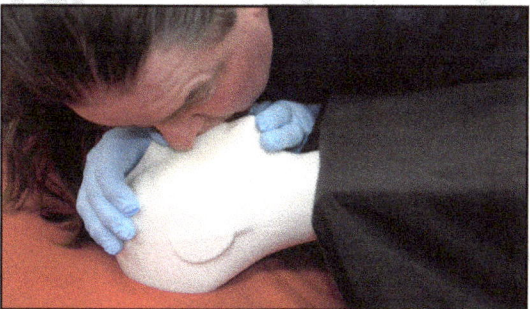

Recheck victim for breathing for 5 seconds. If not breathing continue CPR. "If you determine breaths" keep airway open and monitor victim every 2 minutes for reassessment until medical help arrives.

Remember the chest is a flexible area and having a solid surface to perform compressions is critical. If you find the victim on a sofa, love seat, couch, water bed or other soft area immediately move them to a firm surface.

KEEP LOOKING FOR ANYONE TO HELP WITH CALLING EMS 9-1-1.

CHOKING CONSCIOUS / UNCONSCIOUS RESCUE SKILLS FOR THE CHILD

In all Choking Emergency situations getting Oxygen to the brain is critically important. Without oxygen the brain within 4 - 6 minutes is in danger of brain damage is possible. Within 6 – 8 minutes brain damage is likely. Over 10 minutes irreversible brain damage is certain.

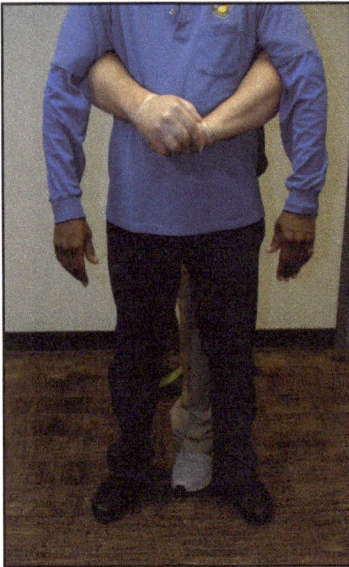

Conscious Choking

Position your feet to stabilize the victim. Rescuer's ankle should be between the victim ankles feet. Rescuer's rear foot should be back enough to brace rescuer and victim.

When placing hands around victims waist just at the belt line, cup the other hand over the inner hand. Inner hand is rolled inward, thumb laid across index finger, not tucked in.
Squeeze inward and upward 5 times.

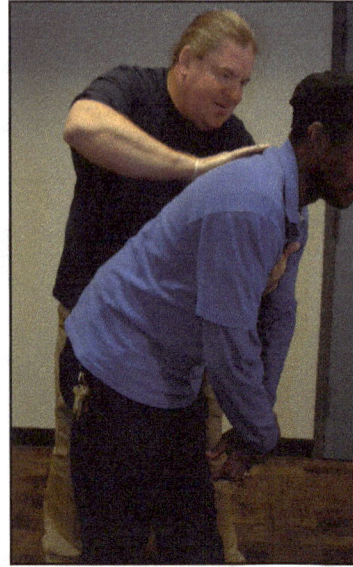

Continue with 5 back blows leaning the victim forward, positioning the head and shoulders lower to expel the object.
One hand should be placed in the victim's upper chest to support the victim.

Using the other hand, heel of the palm continue with 5 blows between the shoulder blades.

If Victims becomes Unconscious start with "Opening the Airway" then "Looking" and "Sweeping the Airway" every time on the Adult/Child.

IF VICTIM BECOMES UNCONSCIOUS

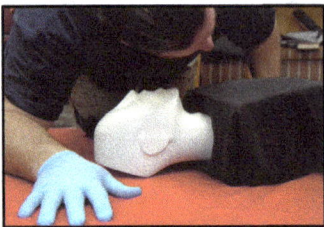

Open, Airway, Use "Index-Pointer finger" to insert into the unconscious victims mouth on side away from you then sweep back in a hooking motion.

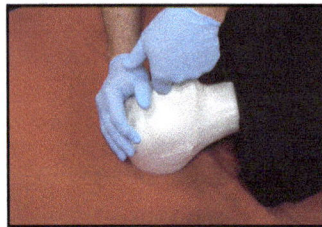

After sweeping the mouth and you see no object or no object was removed begin:

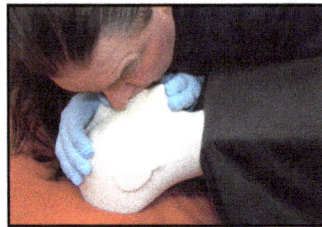

Try and Give 2 breaths. If air did not go in immediately starts chest compressions.

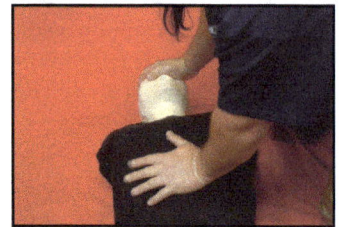

Places your hands on the chest and compress the chest 30 times.

REPEAT the Steps. "Open, Sweep, Breath, Compressions until object comes out or emergency medical help arrives. If victims starts breathing, leave in Shock Position and monitor.

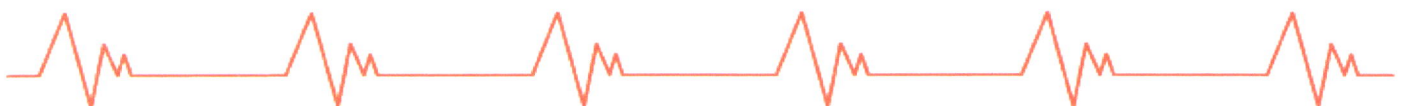

CPR - 6 STEPS FOR INFANTS

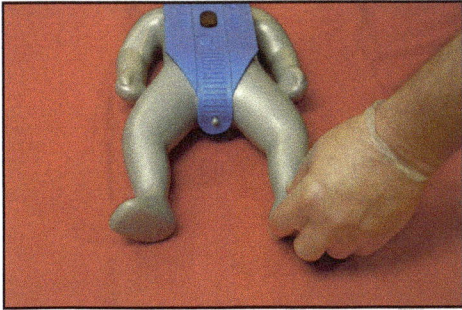

Shake shoulders firmly, "loudly, ask victim, "Are you okay?"

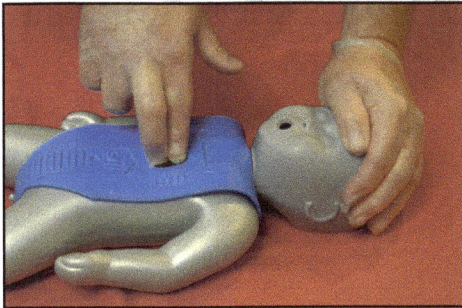

"Quick" Check for Breathing, Look, Listening and Feeling for Breaths. Do Not touch the victim at this point.

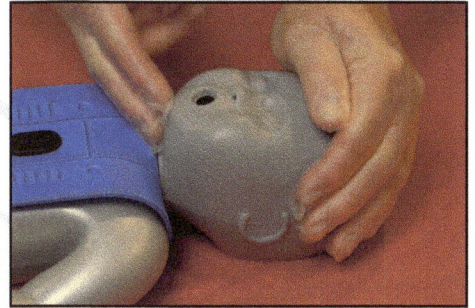

If not Breathing IMMEDIATELY begin CPR, Begin 30 Chest compressions. Place the 2 -3 fingers in the middle of the chest above the sternum just below the nipple line. Compress ½ – 1 inches. (100 compressions per minute is the optimal goal.)

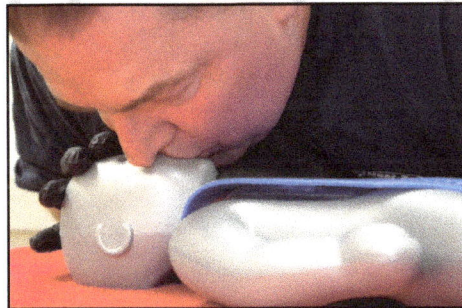

Open the "Air-Way", using Head-Chin-lift method. Never touch the neck.

Place 1 hand on the "lightly on the forehead" and 2 fingers under the boney part of the chin. Tilt chin upward. This takes very little pressure on the infant.

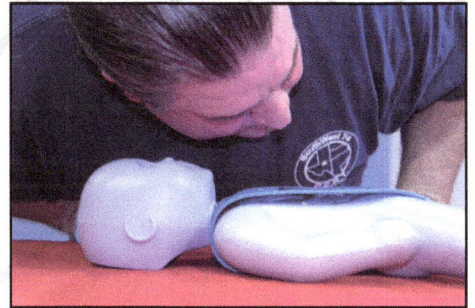

Check Breathing for 5 seconds. If not breathing give 2 breaths, followed immediately with 30 chest compressions performing 5 sets of 30 compressions and 2 breaths. (Using a Breathing Barrier will help to give more oxygen.)

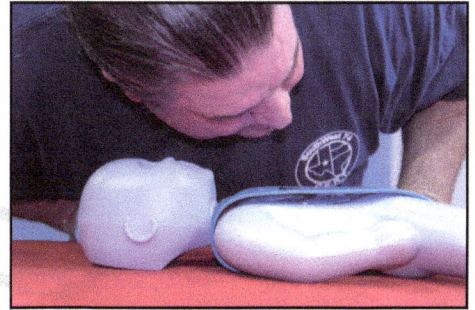

Recheck victim for breathing for 5 seconds. If not breathing continue CPR. "If you determine breaths" keep airway open and monitor victim every 2 minutes for reassessment until

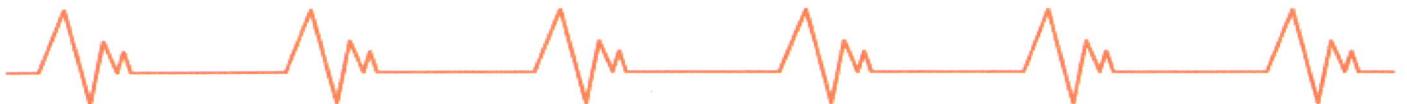

CHOKING CONSCIOUS / UNCONSCIOUS RESCUE SKILLS FOR INFANTS

In all Choking Emergency situations getting Oxygen to the brain is critically important. Without oxygen the brain within 4 - 6 minutes is in danger of brain damage is possible. Within 6 – 8 minutes brain damage is likely. Over 10 minutes irreversible brain damage is certain.

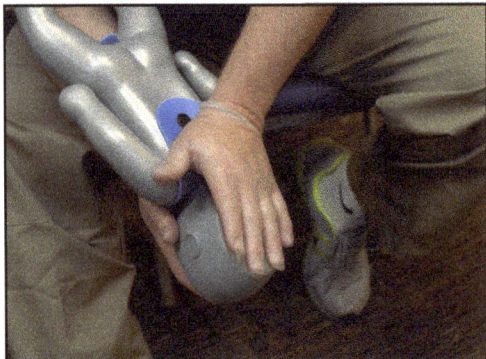

CONSCIOUS CHOKING

After determining Infant obstructed airway, immediately support the Infants head and body with your forearm and place infant face down.

Start with 5 back blows, between shoulders blades.

Always keep head lower than chest during back blows.

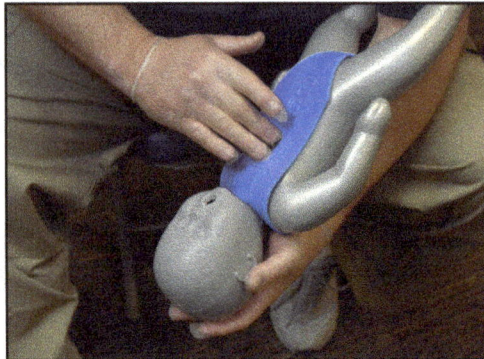

Supporting head and back roll Infant over face up, head lower than chest.

Place 2 middle fingers in the center of chest above the sternum. Press 5 times.

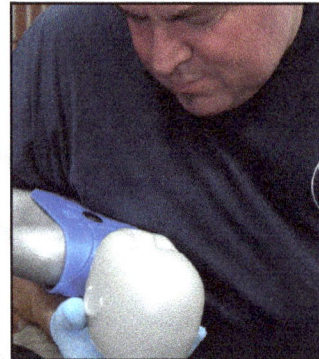

Immediately look into mouth for foreign object.

Infant's mouths are small so look for complete blockage
.
The smallest object can block entire air passage

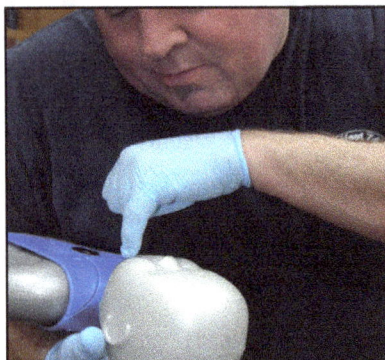

"Only" If object is seen perform finger sweep with little finger.

Finger sweep are in circulation motion. Start with inside jaw furthest away from you and sweep in a loop motion back to sweep object out of mouth. Once object has been removed, give 2 breaths to initiate breathing. Once EMS arrives they will re-evaluate.

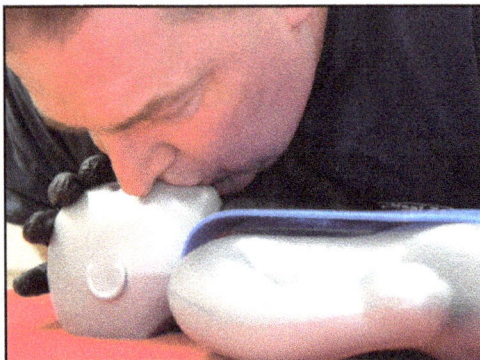

If rescue breathing make sure "seal" your mouth gently over the infants mouth and nose to begin breaths.

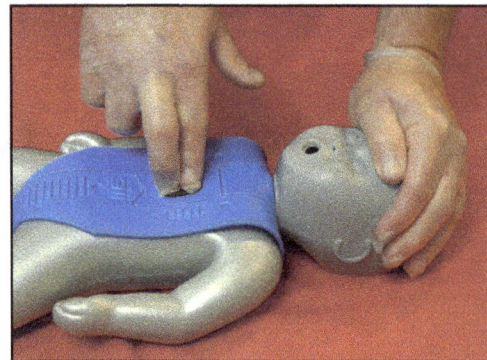

After giving 2 breaths continue with 30 compressions.

REPEAT the Steps. "Open, Sweep, Breath, Compressions until object comes out or emergency medical help arrives. If victims starts breathing, leave in Shock Position and monitor.

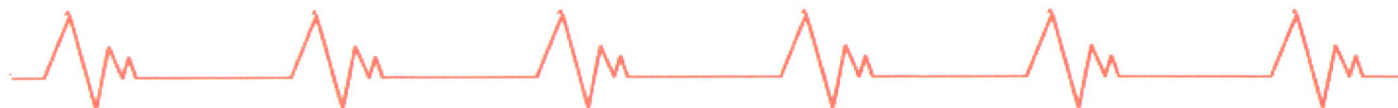

Two Person CPR Adult, Child, and Infant - Professional Health Care Responders

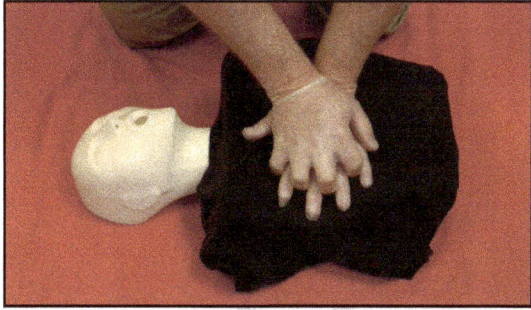

1st Rescuer performs CPR, 30 compressions

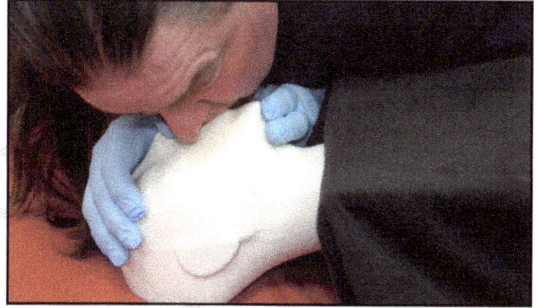

Give 2 breaths, "a second rescuer arrives". Continue giving 30 compressions on Adult while 2nd rescuer places CPR mask on victim. CPR on Child is now 15 compressions.

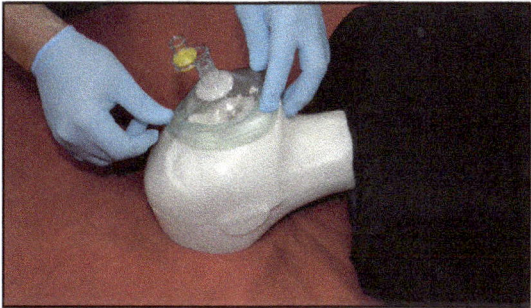

2nd Rescuer starts with 2 breaths, 1st Rescuer continues with 30 chest compressions. 1st Rescuer calls out loud, 26, 27, Ready, Set, Change, they switch. On Child or Infant victim, 15 compressions, 11, 12, Ready, Set, Change.

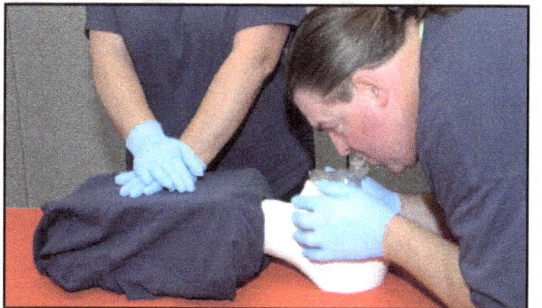

2nd Rescuer places hands on chest and starts compressions while 1st Rescuer gets ready to start with 2 breaths. After 2 minutes, switching sequence is the same.

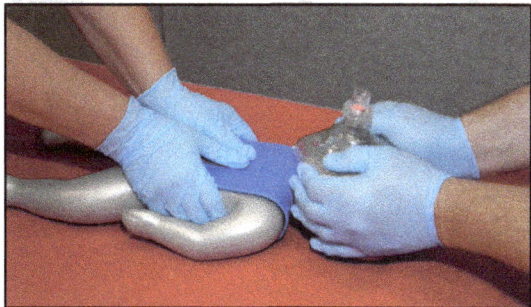

On Infant victim, 1st rescuer places thumbs in center of chest and performs 15 compressions while 2nd rescuer place CPR mask on Infant.

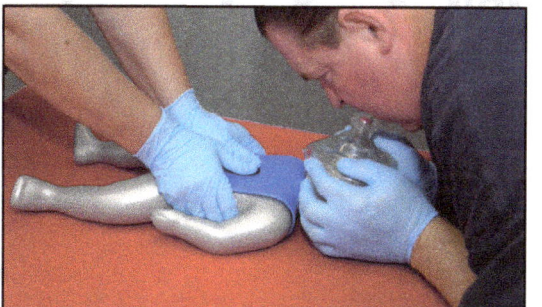

2nd Rescuer performs breaths while 1 st Rescuer continues CPR.

Switch every 2 minutes or at predetermined times.

Remember the chest is a flexible area and having a solid surface to perform compressions is critical. If you find the victim on a sofa, love seat, couch, water bed or other soft area immediately move them to a firm surface.

Recommendations for Stopping CPR: When you see breathing, AED, Unsafe area, Exhausted, Medical help arrives.

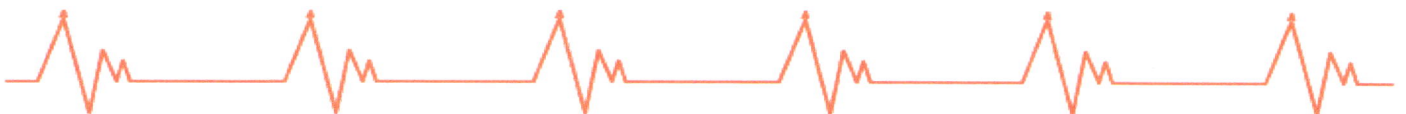

INTENTIONALLY LEFT BLANK

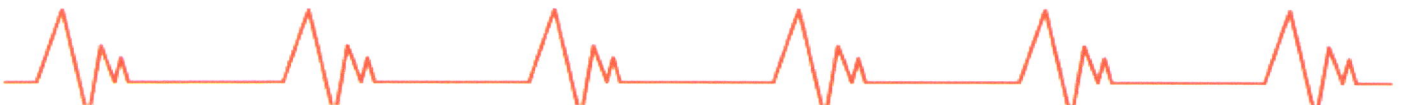

C.P.R.-FACT SHEET ©2015

STEP 1	START STEPS A-C-A-B. (A)rea, (C)ardio Pulmonary Resuscitation-Compressions, (A)irway, (B)reathing	CHECK THE (A)REA/VICTIM FOR ANY DANGERS, AND FOR UNRESPONSIVENESS. CALL FOR ASSISTANCE! Make sure that it is safe for you to approach the injured person. Look for any hidden dangers. Make sure the person that you are checking for injuries are responsive or unresponsive - ADULT or CHILD - Shake shoulders, INFANT - Shake foot firmly. Ask - Are you ok? Look for signs of Life, Motion or Movement. If injured person is unresponsive call out loud for ASSISTANCE! If you are by yourself call 9-1-1 immediately! CONTINUE A.C.A.B'S STEPS
STEP 2	QUICKLY LEAN OVER CHECK FOR (B)REATHS – DETERMINING IF BREATHING, BY LOOKING, LISTENING OR FEELING FOR BREATHS. THIS IS A QUICK CHECK ONLY. IF NOT BREATHING BEGIN COMPRESSIONS (SPECIAL NOTE: If suspected drowning give 2 breaths in this step only)	
STEP 3	GIVE 30 (C)OMPRESSIONS.	PLACE HANDS OR FINGERS IN THE CENTER OF THE CHEST AREA. Victim must be on a hard flat surface. Table, floor, counter top. If victim is on bed, sofa, recliner or couch move victim to floor.

PATIENT	CARDIOPULMONARY RESUSCITATION (CPR)	BREATHS
ADULT 12 years and up	30 Compressions. Compress the chest 1½ – 2 inches Use 2 hands. - One placed on top of the other. Make sure arms are straight over the chest area. Use upper body for compressions. Place hands in center of chest. Inter-lock fingers so that one hand is on top of the other	Give 2 slow full
CHILD 1 year - 12 years	30 Compressions. Compress the chest 1 - 1½ inches. Use 1 hand. Place hand in center of chest. Keep arm straight if possible. Use arm-shoulder for compressions	Give 2 slow regular
INFANT Birth to 1 year	30 Compressions. Compress the chest ½ - 1 inch. Use 2 fingers - place in the middle of the chest.	Give 2 slow small

STEP 4	OPEN THE (A)IRWAY	USE HEAD CHIN / LIFT METHOD. (one hand on forehead, two (2) fingers under bony part of chin). Do not lift the neck, as this may cause further injury if the person has sustained a head, neck, or back injury.
STEP 5	CHECK FOR (B)REATHING 5 SECONDS	If NOT BREATHING, Give victim 2 breathes. Pinch, cover or block the nose. Give 2 slow breaths followed with 30 chest compressions. (5 SETS) Compressions and Breaths. If your injured person is an Adult-give 2 slow FULL breaths, Child-give 2 slow REGULAR breaths, Infant- give 2 slow GENTLE breaths, each breath should be slow but not enough to fill the stomach. IF AIR DID NOT GO IN-REOPEN AIRWAY; IF AIR STILL DID NOT GO IN BEGIN STEPS FOR CHOKING
STEP 6	AFTER 2 MINUTES	Re-check for (B)REATHING 5 SECONDS IF NOT Breathing, continue with CPR-Rescue Breathing combinations until medical help arrives.

REMEMBER C.P.R. ALSO STANDS FOR; "C"-CHECK YOUR VICTIM, "P"-PHONE 9-1-1. "R"-RESCUE VICTIM SAFELY©,

(NEW GUIDELINES FOR CARDIO PULMONARY RESUSCITATION AS PRINTED IN THE JOURNAL OF AMERICAN MEDICAL ASSOCIATION EMERGENCY CARDIAC CARE) VER.2014

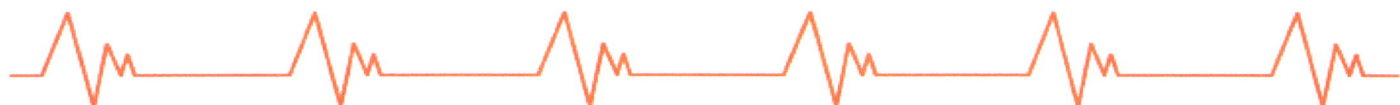

F.A.S.T

F   **FACE:** Ask the person to smile. Does one side of the face droop?

A   **ARMS:** Ask the person to raise both arms. Does one arm drift downward?

S   **SPEECH:** Ask the person to repeat a simple phrase. Is their speech slurred or strange?

T   **TIME:** If you observe any of these signs, call 9-1-1 immediately

By knowing how to quickly evaluate the face, arms, and speech of the person in question, you can help him to get the emergency care he needs for the best possible results.

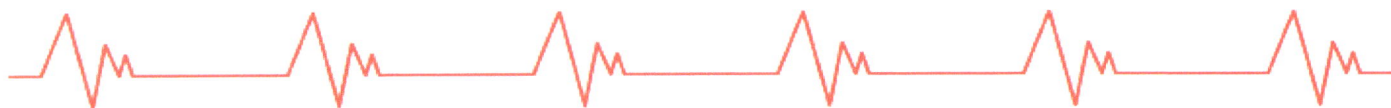

USING AN AED - PRECAUTIONS

WHEN CARDIAC ARREST HAPPENS IMMEDIATELY CALL 9-1-1.

Precautions for Operating an AED:

- "NEVER USE" alcohol to wipe victim's chest as alcohol is flammable.
- "NEVER USE" Adult AED Pads on Children or Infants.
- "USE" appropriate pads as dictated on AED.
- "STAND CLEAR" when AED pads are being placed on victim.
- •"NEVER USE" AED near water or liquids.
- "NEVER USE" AED near a cellular or mobile communications device.
- "NEVER TOUCH" the victim after pads has been placed.

After AED has been attached to victim, turned on, follow automated responses from AED.

BODY HAIR

Some men have excessive chest hair that may result in interference with the AED pads sticking to skin. Remember in this situation to apply pads firmly.

STANDARD PROCEDURES

- Repeated attempts with AED and performing CPR are standard procedures.
- Usually AED's will cycle 3 shocks. Then CPR. Listening to the AED prompts increases better performance.
- For anyone whose heart has stopped chances of survival are greater with the use of combination CPR and AED.
- NEVER leave the victim once AED pads have been placed.
- Once AED has been connected to the victim NEVER remove the pads.
- Professional emergency medical help will issues new directives in care.

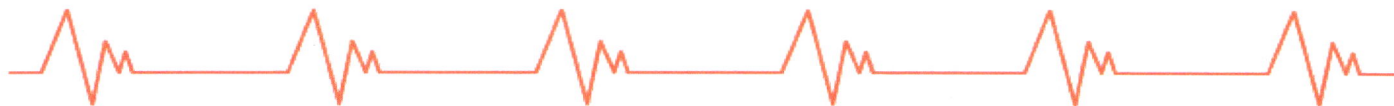

INTENTIONALLY LEFT BLANK

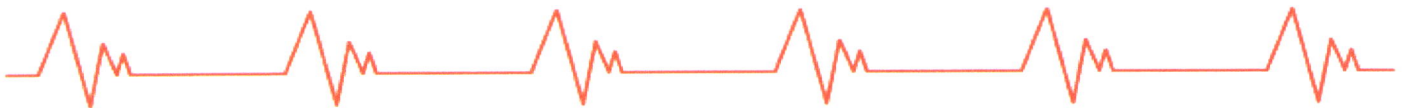

AUTOMATIC EXTERNAL DEFIBRILLATOR (AED) - "QUICK STEPS" ©2014

When performing CPR "if" another RESCUER approaches. They identify themselves and states they can assist. Ask them to retrieve the A.E.D. (Automated External DeAfibrillator).

BELOW ARE AED STEPS FOR ADULTS AND CHILDREN.

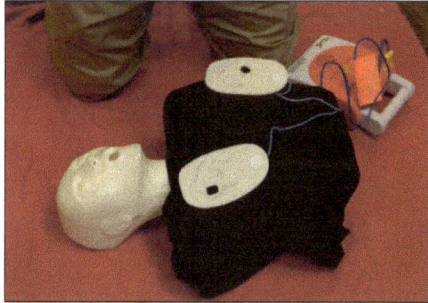

While continuing CPR the second RESCUER opens the A.E.D. Retrieves the electrode pads.

Following instructions on Pads place them on victim.

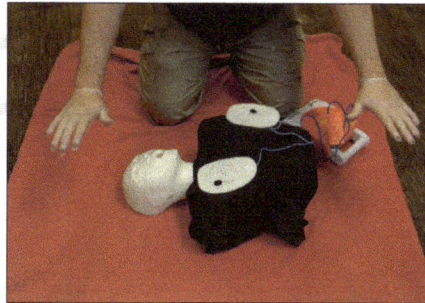

Adult and Children AED pads placement are the same area.

Once Pads are in place rescuer connects to AED and calls out, "Stand Clear".

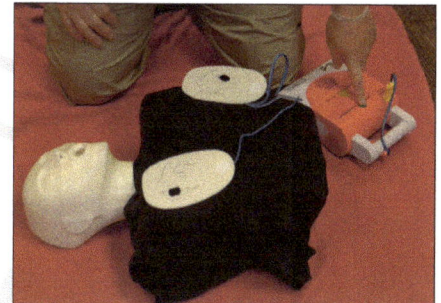

Once area is "Safe" rescuer presses the Start button on AED.

Once the AED is activated follow instructions to the prompts. Continue with CPR

BELOW ARE AED STEPS FOR INFANTS

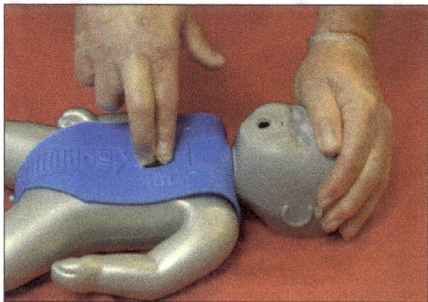

While continuing CPR the second RESCUER opens the A.E.D. Retrieves the electrode pads.

Following instructions on Pads place them on victim.

Continue CPR on Infants until pads are ready to be placed.

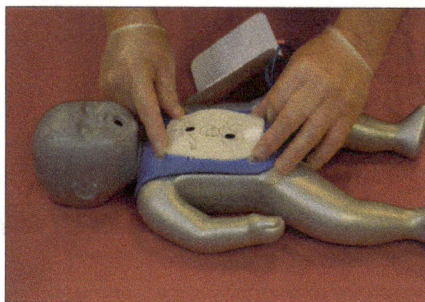

Infants electrode pads are place one in the center chest.

One on the back center (lower right) Once Pads are in place rescuer connects to AED and calls out, "Stand Clear".

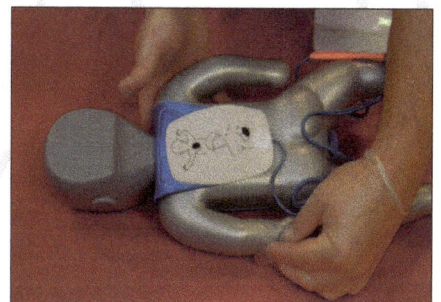

Once area is "Safe" rescuer presses the Start button on AED.

Once the AED is activated follow instructions to the prompts.

AED will advise shock or no shock. Sometimes Responders may not feel pulse but the AED has more sensitive abilities. Continue with AED instructions

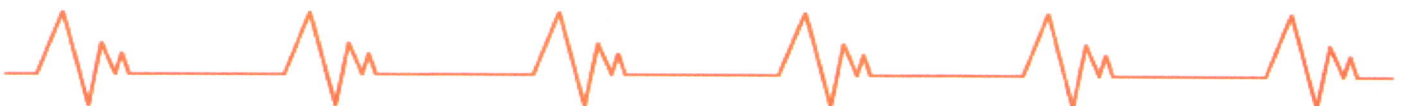

INTENTIONALLY LEFT BLANK

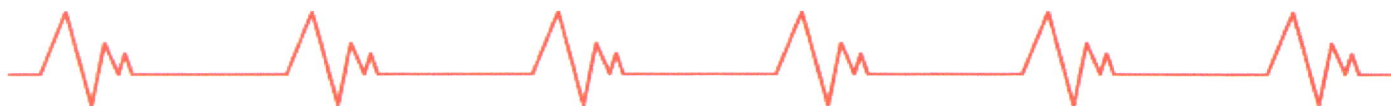

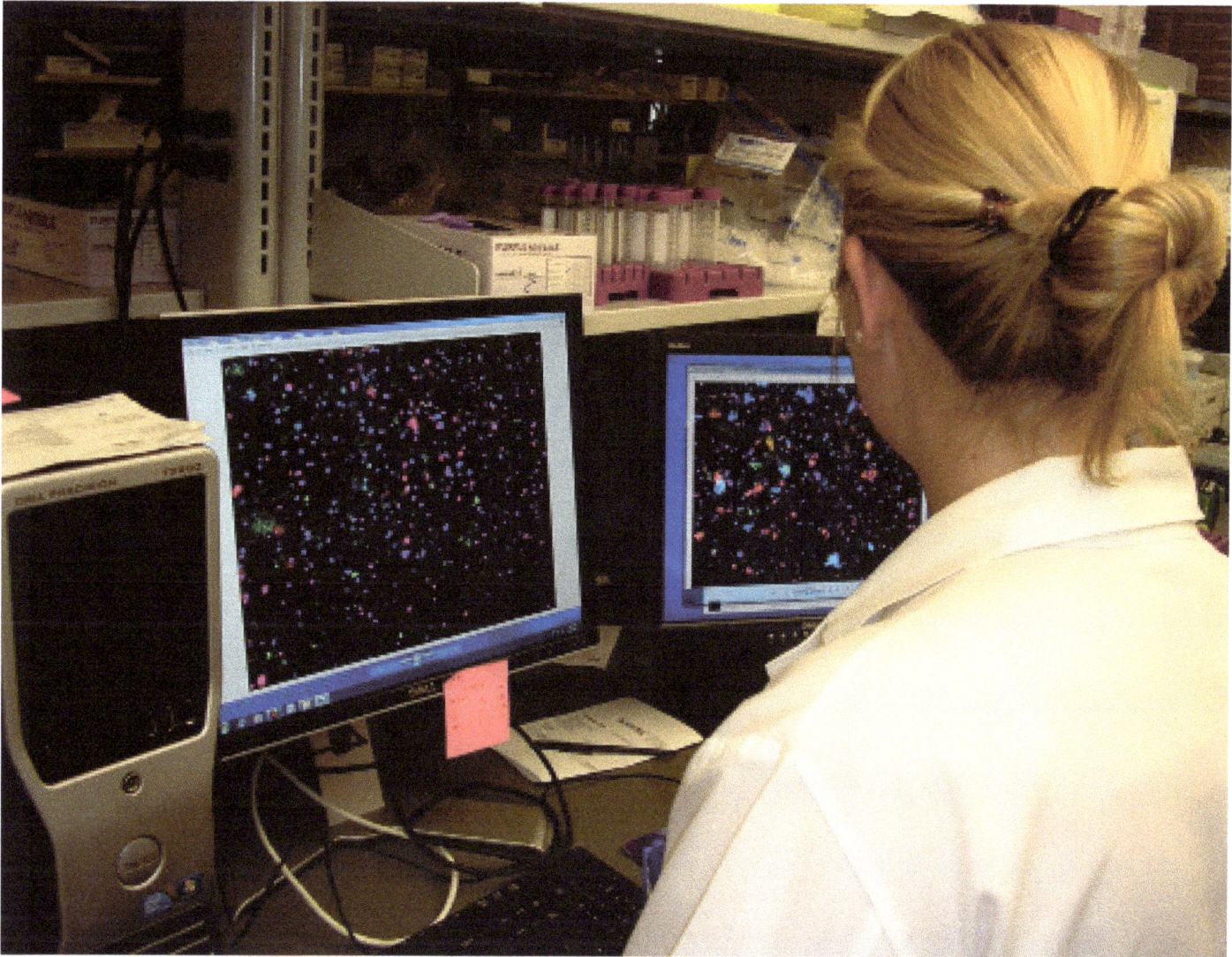

"PATHOLOGY LABORATORY"
PHOTOGRAPHER: DAN SLOAN

INTENTIONALLY LEFT BLANK

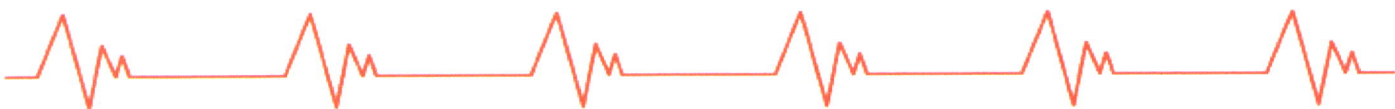

INTRODUCTION

On May 6, 2006, Updated June 2012, the Occupational Safety and Health Administration (OSHA) issued final regulations on job exposure to blood-borne pathogens. These are bacteria and viruses present in human blood and other body fluids that can cause disease in humans. OSHA has determined that employees are at risk when they are exposed on the job to blood and other materials that may cause infections. These materials may contain certain pathogens (germs). These pathogens include hepatitis B virus (HBV) that cause hepatitis B, a serious liver disease, and human immunodeficiency virus (HIV), which causes AIDS.

OSHA has concluded that employers can reduce or remove this hazard from the workplace. This can be done by using a combination of engineering and work practice controls, personal protective clothing and equipment, training, medical surveillance, hepatitis B vaccination, signs and labels, and other provisions.

WHO IS COVERED BY THIS REGULATION?

The regulation defines the range of employees it covers. It includes any employee for whom there is a "reasonable anticipation" of exposure to blood or other materials that could cause infections, while on the job. The hazard of exposure to infectious materials affects employees in many types of jobs. It extends beyond the health care industry.

Employees in the following jobs are covered by this standard if they have on-the-job exposure:

- Employees in health care facilities
- Employees in clinics in factories, schools, and prisons
- Employees assigned to provide emergency first aid
- Employees who handle regulated waste
- Emergency medical technicians, paramedics, and others who provide emergency medical services
- Fire fighters, law enforcement officers, and corrections officers (employees in the private sector, the Federal government, or a state or local government in a state that has an OSHA-approved state plan)
- Linen service employees

The standard does NOT cover any "Good Samaritan" actions that result in exposure to blood or other infectious materials.

WHAT WOULD YOU DO?

A man has collapsed in his office. As the first trained person on the scene, you find the victim bleeding from the mouth and face. Vomit and blood are around him. "His face hit the desk when he fell," a co-worker tells you. He is not breathing. How would you respond? Do you have any concerns about contracting disease?

Some day you may be in a situation such as this, in which you are concerned about disease transmission. You need to understand how infections occur, how they are passed from one person to another, and what you can do to protect yourself and others.

Diseases that can be contracted from people, objects, animals, or insects are often called infectious diseases. Some diseases can be transmitted more easily than others. You need to know how to recognize situations that have the potential for disease transmission and how to protect yourself and others from contracting a disease.

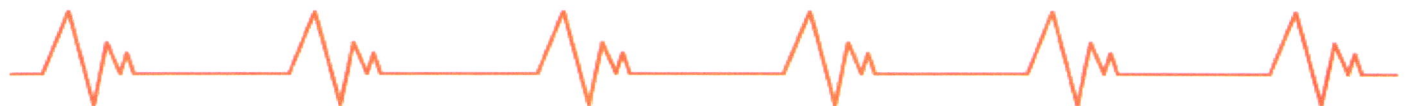

HOW INFECTIONS OCCUR

DISEASE-CAUSING AGENTS

The disease process begins when a pathogen (germ) gets into the body. When pathogens enter the body, they can sometimes overpower the body's defense system and cause illness. This illness is an infection. Most infectious diseases are caused by one of six types of pathogens; the most common are viruses and bacteria.

PATHOGEN	DISEASES AND CONDITIONS THEY CAUSE
Viruses	Hepatitis, measles, mumps, chicken pox, meningitis, rubella, influenza, warts, colds, herpes, shingles, HIV infection including AIDS, genital warts
Bacteria	Tetanus, meningitis, scarlet fever, strep throat, tuberculosis, gonorrhea, syphilis, chlamydia, toxic shock syndrome, Legionnaires' disease, diphtheria, food poisoning
Fungi	Athlete's foot and ringworm
Protozoa	Malaria and dysentery
Rickettsia	Typhus, Rocky Mountain spotted fever
Parasitic Worms	Abdominal pain, anemia, lymphatic vessel blockage, lowered antibody response, respiratory and circulatory complications

Bacteria are everywhere. They do not depend on other organisms for life and can live outside the human body. Most bacteria do not infect humans. Those that do may cause serious illness. Meningitis, scarlet fever, and tetanus are examples of disease caused by bacteria. The body has difficulty fighting infections caused by bacteria. Doctors may prescribe medications called antibiotics that either kill the bacteria or weaken them enough for the body to get rid of them. Commonly used antibiotics include penicillin, erythromycin, and tetracycline.

Unlike bacteria, viruses depend on other organisms to live and reproduce. Viruses cause many diseases, including the common cold. Once they become established within the body, they are difficult to eliminate because very few medications are effective. Antibiotics do not kill or weaken viruses. The body's immune system is the main defense against them.

THE BODY'S NATURAL DEFENSES

The body's immune system is very good at fighting disease. Its basic tools are the white blood cells. Special white blood cells travel around the body identifying invading pathogens. Once they detect a pathogen, these white blood cells gather around it and release antibodies that fight infections.

These antibodies attack the pathogen and weaken or destroy it. Antibodies usually can get rid of the pathogen. However, once inside the body, some pathogens can thrive and, under ideal conditions, overwhelm the immune system. To minimize this possibility, the body depends on the skin for protection to keep pathogens out.

This combination of trying to keep pathogens out of the body and destroying them once they get inside is necessary for good health. Sometimes the body cannot fight off infection. When this occurs, an invading pathogen can become established in the body, causing serious infection. Fever and feeling exhausted often signal that the body is fighting an infection. Other common signals include headache, nausea, and vomiting.

HOW INFECTIONS OCCUR

For a disease to be transmitted, all four of the following conditions must be met:
- A pathogen is present.
- There is enough of the pathogen to cause disease.
- A person is susceptible to the pathogen.
- The pathogen passes through the correct entry site.

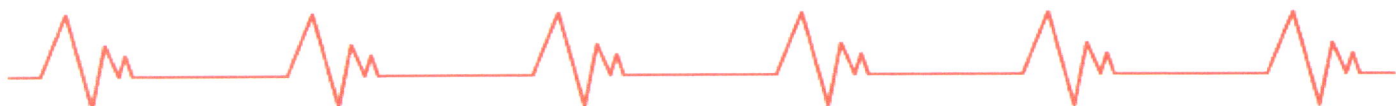

You need to understand these four conditions to understand how infections occur. Think of these conditions as the pieces of a puzzle. All the pieces have to be in place for the picture to be complete. If any one of these conditions is missing, an infection cannot occur.

Pathogens enter the body in four ways:
- *Direct contact
- *Indirect contact
- *Airborne
- *Vector-borne

Not all pathogens can enter the body in all of these ways. For example, certain infections are vector-borne only.

- Direct contact transmission occurs when a person touches body fluids from an infected person.
- Indirect contact transmission occurs when a person touches objects that have touched the blood or another body fluid, such as vomit or saliva, of an infected person. These include soiled dressings, equipment, and work surfaces with which an infected person comes in contact. Sharp objects present a particular risk. If sharp objects have contacted the blood or body fluids of an infected person and are handled carelessly, they can pierce the skin and transmit infection.
- Airborne transmission occurs when a person breathes in droplets that become airborne when an infected person coughs or sneezes. Exposure to these droplets is generally too brief for transmission to take place. If a person is coughing heavily, however, avoid face-to-face contact, if possible.
- Vector transmission occurs when an animal, such as a dog or raccoon, or an insect, such as a tick, transmits a pathogen into the body through a bite. A bite from an infected human also is a vector-borne transmission. The carrier is a vector and passes the infection to another animal or person. Rabies and Lyme disease are transmitted

---

DISEASES THAT CAUSE CONCERN

Some diseases, such as the common cold, are passed from one person to another more easily than others. Although it causes discomfort, the common cold is short-lived and rarely causes serious problems. Other diseases cause more severe problems. Hepatitis B, a liver infection, can last many months. The patient is often seriously ill and slow to recover. Another infection, caused by the human immunodeficiency virus (HIV), destroys the body's ability to fight infection. Both infections can cause prolonged illness or death.

You should be familiar with infections that can have serious consequences if transmitted. These include herpes, meningitis, tuberculosis, hepatitis, and HIV infection, including AIDS.

HERPES

There are several viruses that can cause herpes infections. These viruses cause infections of the skin and mucous membranes. It is very easily passed by direct contact. The herpes virus stays inactive until stimulated. The early stages of herpes may cause headache, sore throat, swelling of the lymph glands, and a general ill feeling. Sometimes swelling occurs around the lips and mouth where small sores like blisters may form. These are commonly called cold sores.

In a more serious form of herpes, sores appear on the face, neck, and shoulders. Another form of herpes causes sores in the genital area. Since antibiotics do not work against viruses, the infection runs its course and becomes inactive for a while. It then flares up again. Herpes is usually transmitted through direct contact with sores. It enters through an opening in the skin or through mucous membranes, such as those in the mouth or eyes. You should avoid unprotected contact with people who have active herpes.

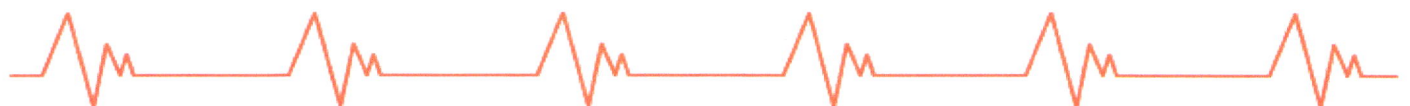

Meningitis

Meningitis is a severe infection of the covering of the brain and spinal cord. Either viruses or bacteria can cause it. It is easily transmitted by direct, indirect, and airborne means.

You can get the viral form of meningitis from contaminated food and water. Bacterial meningitis can be transmitted through the mucus in the nose and mouth. The germs might be passed if an infected person coughs near your face or if you come in direct contact with the person's mucus. You could get bacterial meningitis from unprotected rescue breathing.

Although meningitis is more common in infants and young children, adults are not immune. The first signals are often respiratory infections, sore throat, stiff neck, rash, nausea, and vomiting. An infected person may quickly become seriously ill. In its advanced stages, a person may become unconscious. Meningitis, if treated early, is rarely fatal.

Tuberculosis

Tuberculosis most often affects the respiratory system. The bacteria that cause it live in the lungs. Infection occurs mainly from inhaling droplets that contain the bacteria. The disease causes weight loss, night sweats, occasional fever, and a general feeling of tiredness. The signals often develop gradually so people may not notice the early stages. People who do not know they have tuberculosis may even remain in fairly good health for a long time before they rapidly become ill. If the victim is not coughing, and you have no contact with material coughed up by the patient, you are unlikely to be infected.

Hepatitis

Hepatitis is an inflammation of the liver. The most common forms of hepatitis are caused by alcohol abuse, drugs, or other chemicals and cannot be transmitted. Viruses, however, also can cause hepatitis. The two most common types of viral hepatitis are type A and type B.

Hepatitis A is also called infectious hepatitis. It is common in children. It is often transmitted by contact with food or other products soiled by the stool of an infected person. Parents may get the disease from their children by changing diapers. Shellfish and water containing the virus also can transmit hepatitis A.

People with hepatitis A at first feel as if they have flu. Later, their skin may become a yellowish color, a condition called jaundice. Hepatitis A usually does not have serious consequences.

Hepatitis B is a severe liver infection caused by the hepatitis B virus. Hepatitis B is primarily transmitted by sexual contact and blood-to-blood contact from transfusions, needle sticks, cuts, scrapes, sores, and skin irritations. Hepatitis B has also been found in other body fluids such as saliva.

Hepatitis B is not transmitted by casual contact, such as shaking hands. It is not transmitted by indirect contact with objects like drinking fountains or telephones. Your risk most often occurs in unprotected direct or indirect contact with infected blood.

The signals of hepatitis B are similar to the flu like signals of hepatitis A. Hepatitis B infections can be fatal. The disease may be in the body for up to six months before signals appear. The person may then overlook the flu like signals. Some people can even develop chronic hepatitis after recovering from the early signals.

Non A-Non B Hepatitis is a third form of hepatitis. If a virus cannot be clearly identified as hepatitis A or hepatitis B, it is

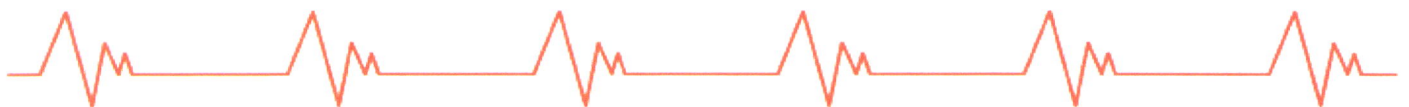

HOW DISEASES ARE TRANSMITTED

DISEASE	SIGNS & SYMPTOMS	MODE OF TRANSMISSION	INFECTIVE MATERIAL
Herpes	Lesions, general ill feeling, sore throat	Direct contact	Broken skin, mucous membranes
Meningitis	Respiratory illness, sore throat, nausea, vomiting	Airborne, direct and indirect contact	Food and water, mucus
Tuberculosis	Weight loss, night sweats, occasional fever, general ill feeling	Airborne, direct contact	Mucus, broken skin
Hepatitis	Flu like, jaundice	Direct and indirect contact	Blood, saliva, semen, feces, food, water, other products
HIV/AIDS	Fever, night sweats, weight loss, chronic diarrhea, severe fatigue, shortness of breath, swollen lymph nodes, lesions	Direct and indirect contact	Blood, semen, vaginal fluid

HIV/AIDS

AIDS (acquired immunodeficiency syndrome) is a result of a weakened immune system. It is caused by HIV (human immunodeficiency virus). This virus attacks white blood cells and destroys the body's ability to fight infection. The infections that strike people whose immune systems are weakened by HIV or other conditions include severe pneumonia and fungal infections of the mouth and esophagus. HIV-infected people may also develop Kaposi's sarcoma and other unusual cancers.

People infected with HIV may not feel or look sick. A blood test, however, can detect the HIV antibody. When the infected person shows signs of having certain infections or cancers, he or she may be diagnosed as having AIDS. The infections can cause severe fatigue, fever, night sweats, unexplained weight loss, chronic diarrhea, shortness of breath, swollen lymph nodes, and skin lesions. In the advanced stages, AIDS is a very serious condition. Victims get life-threatening infections.

It is important to remember the following points about the transmission of HIV:

- HIV cannot be spread through casual contact.
- The virus that causes HIV infection is easily killed by alcohol, chlorine bleach, and other common disinfectants. You cannot bring a dead virus back to life by adding water.
- HIV is known to be transmitted only through exposure to infected blood, semen, vaginal secretions, or (rarely) breast milk.

This can occur by:

- Having unprotected sex with an infected partner, male or female.
- Being exposed to blood through use of soiled equipment or supplies, needle stick injuries, or blood splashed on mucous membranes or broken skin. (The risk of getting infected through a blood transfusion or blood product is very low since 1985.)
- Sharing needles or syringes for street drugs, steroids, or ear piercing.
- Being infected as an unborn child or shortly after birth by an infected mother.

CHILDHOOD DISEASES

Most people have been immunized against the common childhood diseases such as measles and mumps. An immunization is the introduction of a substance that contains specific weakened or killed pathogens into the body. The body's immune system then builds a resistance to the specific infection.

No immunization exists, however, for chicken pox (varicella). The varicella infection causes fever and "pox" (blister like sores on the skin). Once you have had chicken pox, it is unlikely that you will contract the disease again.

You might not have been immunized against some of the childhood diseases. If you are not sure about which immuniza-

PROTECTING YOURSELF FROM DISEASE TRANSMISSION

THE EXPOSURE CONTROL PLAN

Preventing infectious disease begins with preparation and planning. An Exposure Control Plan is an important step in removing or reducing employee exposure to blood and other possibly infectious materials. The Exposure Control Plan is the way in which an employer creates a system to protect its employees from infection. It is a key provision of the OSHA standard. The plan requires the employer to identify who will receive training, protective equipment, and vaccination.

An Exposure Control Plan should contain the following elements:

- Exposure determination
-
- The schedule and method of implementing other parts of the OSHA standard, (i.e., ways of meeting the requirements and record keeping)
-
- The procedures for evaluating details of an exposure incident.

Exposure determination is one of the key elements of the Exposure Control Plan. It includes identifying and making a written record of jobs where exposure to blood can occur. The determination should be made without regard to using personal protective equipment.

The Exposure Control Plan should be placed where employees can easily use it and must be updated each year or more often if changes in exposure occur.

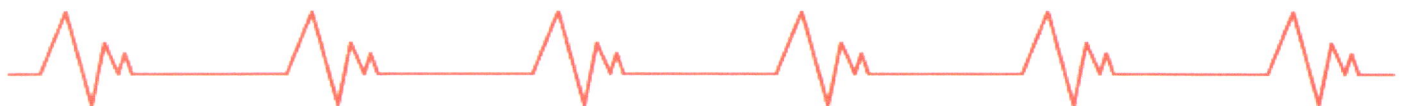

IMMUNIZATIONS

Preventing infectious diseases begins with maintaining good health and always practicing good personal hygiene such as washing hands frequently. You should also be immunized against several diseases. The following immunizations are recommended:

- DPT (Diphtheria, pertussis, tetanus)
- Polio
- Hepatitis B
- MMR (measles, mumps, rubella)
- Influenza
-

Check with your doctor to see whether you need any boosters to keep your immunizations up to date.

The OSHA standard requires that an employer make the hepatitis B vaccination series available to all employees who have job exposure to blood or other body fluids. It also requires post-exposure evaluation and follow-up to all employees who have an exposure incident.

The employer shall make sure that all medical evaluations and procedures, including the hepatitis B vaccination series and post-exposure evaluation and follow-up are:

- Made available at no cost to the employee.
- Made available to employees at a reasonable time and place.
- Provided by or under the supervision of a licensed physician or health care professional. (People getting vaccinations should be carefully watched for at least thirty minutes after injection. Approximately 10% of all individuals will have an allergic reaction to the vaccine.)
- Provided according to the current recommendations of the U.S. Public Health Office.

OSHA has also added special considerations for employees who provide first aid for incidents occurring in the workplace. OSHA believes there is a low risk of exposure for these first aiders. The option of post-exposure prevention measures, including hepatitis B vaccination within 24 hours of exposure, is now available. OSHA believes that this option will minimize the risk to employees and lessen demands on limited supplies of the vaccine.

This option applies to employees whose routine work assignment does not include administering first aid. It does not apply to employees who provide first aid at a first aid station, clinic or dispensary, or to health care, emergency response or public safety personnel expected to provide first aid in the course of their work.

OSHA considers the selection of this option a technical violation of the standard, but does not impose any penalty on the employer. However, the following conditions must be met:

- The Exposure Control Plan must include reporting procedures for first aid incidents involving exposure. The procedures must ensure that incidents are reported before the end of the shift in which they occur.
- Reports of first aid incidents must include the names of all first aiders involved and the details of the incident. The report must also include the date and time of the incident and if an exposure incident has occurred.
- Exposure reports must be included on lists of first aid incidents. They must be readily available to employees and provided to OSHA on request.
- First aid providers must be trained under the blood-borne pathogens standard that covers the reporting procedure specifics.
- All first aiders who provide assistance in any incident involving blood or other potentially infectious materials, regardless of whether a specific exposure incident occurs, must be offered the full Hepatitis B vaccination series. This immunization should be offered as soon as possible, but in no event later than 24 hours following exposure. If an exposure incident occurs, other post-exposure follow-up procedures must be initiated immediately.

UNIVERSAL PRECAUTIONS

Sometimes we might like to vary the level of protection we use based on what a person looks like, the circumstances surrounding the incident, or where he or she is at the time of the incident. However, the world is not that simple. Very often you will not know the health status of the people you work with or care for. The one time you stop being careful may be the very time that you become infected by someone who does not fit into your notion of people who are likely to be infected. Each time you prepare to provide care, you must follow basic universal precautions. Universal Precautions include four areas:

- Protective equipment
- Personal hygiene
- Engineering and work practice controls
- Equipment cleaning and disinfecting.

Protective equipment includes all equipment and supplies that keep you from direct contact with infected materials. These include disposable gloves, gowns, masks and shields, protective eyewear, and mouthpieces and resuscitation devices. To minimize your risk of contracting or transmitting an infectious disease, follow these guidelines for the use of protective equipment.

- Wear disposable (single-use) gloves, when it is possible you will contact blood or body fluids. This may happen directly through contact with a victim or indirectly through contact with soiled clothing or other personal articles.
- Remove gloves by turning them inside out, beginning at the wrist and peeling them off. When removing the second glove, do not touch the soiled surfaces with your bare hand. Hook the inside of the glove at the wrist and peel the glove off. [See below]
- Discard gloves that are peeling, discolored, torn, or punctured.
- Do not clean or reuse disposable gloves.
- Avoid handling items such as pens, combs, or radios (yours or another person's) when wearing soiled gloves.
- Change gloves when you contact different victims.
- Wear protective coverings, such as a mask, eyewear, and gown, whenever you are likely to contact blood or other body fluids that may splash.
- Cover any cuts, scrapes, or skin irritations you may have with protective clothing and/or bandages.
- Use breathing devices such as disposable resuscitation masks and airway devices.

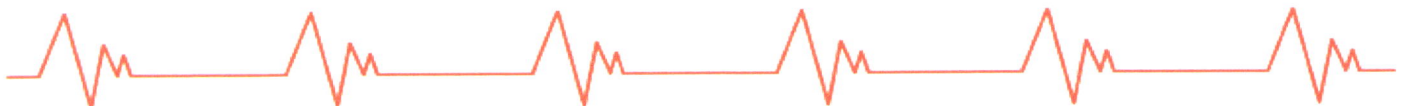

RECOMMENDED PROTECTIVE EQUIPMENT AGAINST HIV AND HBV TRANSMISSION IN PRE-HOSPITAL SETTINGS

TASK OR ACTIVITY	DISPOSABLE GLOVES	GOWN	MASK	PROTECTIVE EYEWEAR
Bleeding Control With Spurting Blood	Yes	Yes	Yes	Yes
Bleeding Control With Minimal Bleeding	Yes	No	No	No
Emergency Childbirth	Yes	Yes	Yes, If Splashing Is Likely	Yes, if splashing is likely
Helping With Intravenous (Iv) Line	Yes	No	No	No
Oral/Nasal Suctioning Manually Clearing Airway	Yes	No	No, Unless Splashing Is Likely	No, unless splashing is likely
Handling And Cleaning Contaminated Equipment And Clothing	Yes	NO, UNLESS SOILING IS LIKELY	No	No

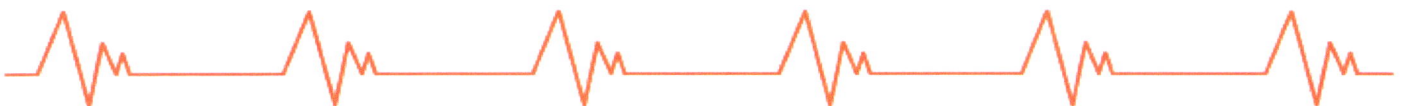

ENGINEERING CONTROLS & PERSONAL HYGIENE

Engineering controls are controls that isolate or remove the hazard from the workplace. Engineering controls include puncture-resistant containers for sharp equipment and mechanical needle recapping devices. To ensure that they work well, engineering controls should be examined and maintained or replaced on a regular basis. Once put in place, engineering controls should be maintained and replaced periodically.

Work place controls reduce the likelihood of exposure by changing the way a task is carried out. The protection provided by work practice controls is based on the way an employer and employee behave rather than on a physical device.

Your personal hygiene habits are as important in preventing infection as any equipment you might use. These habits and practices can prevent any materials that might have gotten through the protective equipment from staying in contact with your body. Following certain guidelines for personal hygiene can greatly cut down your risk of contracting or transmitting an infectious disease.

Engineering controls and work practice controls are established to ensure good industrial hygiene. Following certain guidelines for engineering controls and work practice controls can greatly cut down your risk of getting or transmitting an infectious disease.

- Avoid needle stick injuries by not trying to bend or recap any needles.
- If a procedure requires the recapping of a needle, use mechanical devices or one-handed techniques to recap or remove contaminated needles.
- Place sharp items (needles, scalpel blades, etc.) in puncture-resistant, leak proof, labeled containers.
- Prohibit mouth pipetting or suctioning of blood or other potentially infectious materials.
- Perform all procedures in such a way that cuts down on splashing, spraying, splattering and producing droplets of blood or other potentially infectious materials.
- Remove blooded soiled protective clothing as soon as possible.
- Clean and disinfect all equipment and work surfaces possibly soiled by blood or other body fluids.
- Wash your hands thoroughly with soap and water immediately after providing care. Use a utility or restroom sink, not one in a food preparation area.
- Avoid eating, drinking, smoking, applying cosmetics or lip balm, handling contact lenses, and touching the mouth, nose, or eyes in work areas where an exposure to
- Infectious materials may occur.

It is important to clean and disinfect equipment to prevent infections. Handle all soiled equipment, supplies, or other materials with great care until they are properly cleaned and disinfected. Place all disposable items, which are contaminated in labeled containers. Place all soiled clothing in properly marked plastic bags for disposal or washing.

To disinfect equipment soiled with blood or body fluids, wash thoroughly with a solution of common household chlorine bleach and water. Approximately ¼ cup of bleach per gallon of water is enough. Surfaces, such as floors, woodwork, ambulance and automobile seats, and countertops, must be cleaned of any soil you can see before using a bleach solution.

Wash and dry protective clothing and work uniforms according to the manufacturer's instructions. Scrub soiled boots, leather shoes, and other leather goods, such as belts, with soap, a brush, and hot water.

If an incident occurs that creates disposable waste or soiled laundry, the employer should provide containers to store the materials until they are disposed of or laundered. The containers must have warnings labels or signs, such as "biohazard", to eliminate or minimize exposure of employees. In addition, the employer must provide training to ensure that all employees understand and avoid the hazard.

The OSHA standard requires that the employer keep the work area in a clean and sanitary condition. The employer is re-

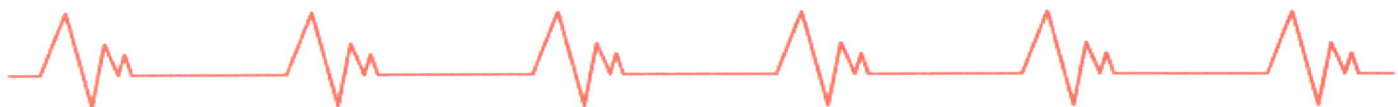

quired to develop and put into action a written schedule for cleaning and decontamination at the work site. The schedule should be based on the location in the facility, the type of surface to be cleaned, the type of soil present, and the task or procedures being done.

In addition, the employer has a responsibility to have a plan in place to deal with any spill that might occur. The plan should include a system to report the spill, and the action taken to resolve the spill. It should also include a list of employees responsible for containment, instructions for cleanup, and the final disposition of the spill.

The first step in dealing with a spill is containment. Spill containment units designed for hazardous materials are sold and work very well. However, any absorbent material, such as paper towels, can be used if the material is disposed of properly.

The steps for spill management are as follows:

- Wear gloves and other appropriate personal protective equipment when cleaning spills.
- Clean up spills immediately, or as soon as possible after the spill occurs.
- If the spill is mixed with sharp objects such as broken glass and needles, do not pick these up with your hands. Use tongs, broom and dustpan, or two pieces of cardboard.
- Dispose of the absorbent material used to collect the spill in a labeled biohazard container.
- Flood the area with disinfectant solution, and allow it to stand for at least twenty minutes.
- Use paper towels to absorb the solution, and put the towels in the biohazard container.

Following these universal precautions will usually remove at least one of the four conditions necessary for disease transmission. Remember, if only one condition is missing, infection will not occur.

IF EXPOSURE OCCURS

If you suspect you have been exposed to an infectious disease, wash any area of contact as quickly as possible and write down what happened. Exposures usually involve contact with potentially infectious blood or other fluids through a needle stick, broken or scraped skin, or the mucous membranes of the eyes, nose, or mouth. Inhaling potentially infected airborne droplets also may be an exposure. Most employers have protocols (standardized methods) for reporting infectious disease exposure.

Protocols should include the following elements:

- List of events included in the protocol
- List of immediate actions to be taken by exposed employee to reduce the chances of infection
- When or how quickly the employee should report the exposure incident
- Where and to whom the employee should report the exposure incident
- Which forms the employee should complete
- Directions for investigating the incident
- Medical follow-up that would include post-exposure vaccination.

If you think you have been exposed to an infectious disease, it is your responsibility to notify your supervisor immediately. A test may be done to see if the material was in fact infected. But even before a disease is confirmed, you should receive medical evaluation, counseling, and post-exposure care, such as the Hepatitis B vaccine. Your supervisor or medical personnel is responsible for notifying any other personnel who might have been exposed. If your system does not have a designated physician or nurse at a local hospital for follow-up care, see your personal physician.

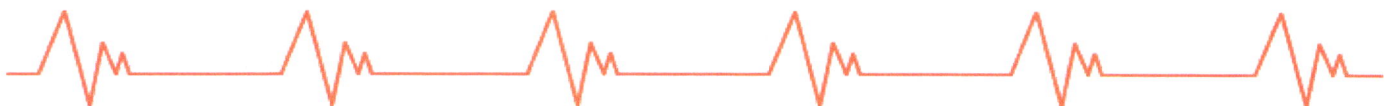

SUMMARY

Although the body's natural defense system defends well against disease, pathogens can still enter the body and sometimes cause infection. These pathogens can be transmitted in four ways:

- By direct contact with an infected person
- By indirect contact with a soiled object
- By inhaling air exhaled by an infected person
- Through a bite from an infected animal, insect, or even a person.

Infectious diseases that you should be aware of include hepatitis, herpes, meningitis, tuberculosis, and HIV infection, including AIDS. You should know how the diseases are transmitted and take appropriate measures to protect yourself from them. Remember that the four conditions of infection must be present for a disease to be transmitted.

The Occupational Safety and Health Administration (OSHA) have issued regulations for on-the-job exposure to blood-borne pathogens. The agency has determined that employees face a significant risk as a result of on-the-job exposure to blood and other potentially infectious materials because they may contain blood-borne pathogens. OSHA concludes that this hazard can be reduced or removed using a combination of engineering and work practice controls, personal protective clothing and equipment, training, medical surveillance, hepatitis B vaccination, signs and labels, and other provisions.

The OSHA regulation defines the range of employees covered by the standard, and it sets forth certain requirements that employers must meet to maintain work sites in a clean and sanitary condition.

The regulations on blood-borne pathogens have placed specific responsibilities on employers for protection of employees that include:

- Identifying positions or tasks covered by the standard
- Creating an Exposure Control Plan to minimize the possibility of exposure
- Using work practices, such as following universal precautions to minimize the possibility of infection
- Using engineering controls, such as puncture-resistant containers for sharp objects, to minimize the possibility of infection
- Creating a system for easy identification of soiled material and its disposal
- Developing a system of annual training for all covered employees
- Offering the opportunity for employees to get counseling and medical care such as the Hepatitis B vaccination at no cost
- Establishing clear procedures to follow for reporting an exposure
- Creating a system of record keeping that includes updates in protocols and Exposure Control Plans, employee training, employee medical records, and follow-up.

Following OSHA guidelines, especially the universal precautions, greatly decreases your risk of contracting or transmitting an infectious disease. If you suspect you have been exposed to such a disease, always document it or notify your supervisor and other involved personnel. Seek medical help and participate in any follow-up procedures.

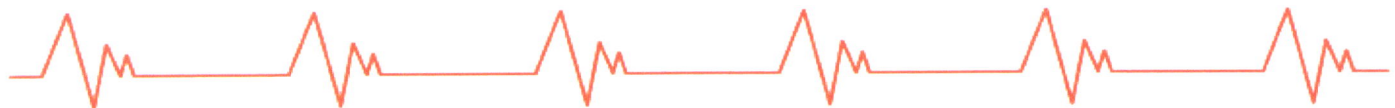

ATTRIBUTIONS AND PERMISSIONS

Photo of Diamondback Rattlesnake (Cortalus atrox) by Clinton & Charles Robertson from Del Rio, Texas & College Station, TX, USA, used under the terms of the Creative Commons Generic license.

GLOSSARY

Abdomen	The belly; Below the diaphragm and above the pelvis	Airway blockage (obstruction)	Objects or conditions that prevent normal air flow to the lungs
Abdominal Thrusts	Technique used to describe forceful motions to remove air from the body	Amputation	Removal of a part of the body
Abrasion	Part of the body that has been scraped, rubbed or torn; Referred to as a "Strawberry" in sports	Anaphylaxis / Anaphylactic	A severe, potentially life-threatening allergic reaction that may result in restricted or blocked airway and shock
Absorbed poison	A toxic substance taken into the body through unbroken skin	Anaphylaxis treatment	Medications used to off-set the direct allergic reaction; Epipen or anti-histamines
ACLS	Advanced Cardiovascular Life Support - Techniques for the urgent treatment of cardiac arrest, stroke and other life-threatening medical emergencies	Anatomic splint	Using two parts of the body to immobilize another injured part, i.e. fingers
		Aneurysm	Enlargement of an artery caused by a weakening of the artery wall; May be caused by trauma, muscle weakness, or disease
Adult	Age 13 years and up		
Advance Directives	Written documentation that describes desired treatment or care	Angina	Upper chest pain normally associated with inadequate blood flow to the heart, i.e. heart attack
AED	Automated External Defibrillator - A portable device that checks the heart rhythm and can send an electric shock to the heart to try to restore a normal rhythm		
		Anterior	The front (face side) of the body
		Antibiotics	Specific medicines often used to fight bacterial infections
AIDS	Acquired Immunodeficiency Syndrome - Transmissible disease of the immune system caused by HIV; Last stage of HIV infection	Antibodies	A protein made by the body that detects and helps destroy invaders, like bacteria and viruses
		Anxiety	A feeling of worry, nervousness, unease, or fear; The source of the symptoms is not always known
Airborne transmission	Disease causing bacteria or viruses that travel from one body to another on dust particles or small moisture droplets formed by sneeze, cough, laugh, or exhale		
		Arm	Extremity from shoulder to hand
Airway	The passage by which air reaches a person's lungs.	Arteries	Tubes that carry blood FROM the heart to all parts of the body

Aspiration	Foreign material entering airway to lungs	Brachial Artery	The major blood vessel of the (upper) arm; located on the body-side of the arm between armpit and elbow
Assessment	Immediate determination of injuries	Brachial Pulse	Located in the upper inside of the arm
Asthma	Respiratory condition that restricts normal breathing	Brain	Controls the sensory and nervous system of the body
Asystole	Complete stop of all electrical activity of the heart	Breathing apparatus	BVM, CPR Mask, Non-Rebreather mask, made to assist in respiration delivery
Atherosclerosis / Arteriosclerosis	Cardiovascular Disease restricting blood flow to the heart and body	Burn	Injury to the body or skin tissue by heat, electricity, chemicals or radiation
Aura	The unusual feeling or sensation before a seizure: Smell, taste, sound, or panic to get to safety	BVM	Bag Valve Mask, large volume respiration assistance, may be used with or without O2
Avulsion	Torn or open part of the wound	Capillaries	Small blood vessels that transfer oxygen and nutrition, remove waste products
Bacteria	Single cell microorganism that causes infections	Carbon Dioxide	Tasteless, odorless gas, by-product of respiration
Bag Valve Mask	BVM - Large volume respiration assistance, may be used with or without O2	Cardiac Arrest	Heart stops or beats in an irregular rhythm, too weakly to transfer blood to the arteries
Bee Sting	More likely than others to cause allergic or toxic reactions	Carotid Artery	Located either side of the neck, towards the mid center of the neck, Provides blood to the head / brain
Biological Death	Death of the brain from lack of oxygen about 10 - 12 minutes after breathing and blood circulation stop	CDC	Centers for Disease Control and Prevention, the US agency charged with tracking and investigating public health trends, located in Atlanta, Georgia
Bite, Human	normally 6 - 8 teeth punctures		
Bite, Snake	Sharp, low body areas vulnerable	Cells	Basic structure of living tissues; The smallest structural and functional unit of an organism
Bite, Tick	Seasonal, several species are disease carriers		
Blanch Test	Squeezing of the tip of a finger or body skin and release to observe color flow refill of veins	Cervical collar	Rigid device to minimize the movement of the neck
Blood	The red liquid that flows through the bodies of people; carries oxygen in cells; 1 pint of blood per 25 pounds of body weight	Chest Thrusts	Forced compression on the chest to help remove a foreign object
Blood Pressure	Force or pressure of blood through the circulatory system	Child	Age 1 year to 13 years
Blood Volume	Total amount of blood circulating		
Bone	Dense tissue, calcium, forms the skeleton		

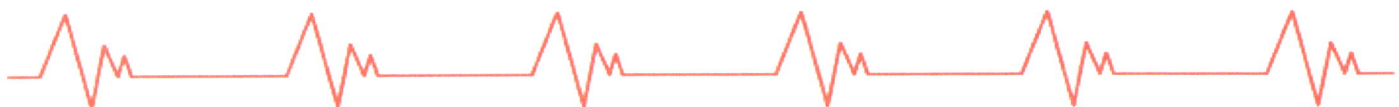

Circulatory system	Body organs (heart, blood vessels, etc.) to carry oxygen through the body	Defibrillator	Mechanical device that delivers an electric shock to the heart
CISD	Critical Incident Stress Debriefing - A crisis intervention process	Diastolic	Arterial blood pressure during the time between heartbeats
Clinical Death	Both Heart and breathing stop	DirectContact Transmission	Physical (by touching or contact with body fluids) transfer of microorganisms from an infected person to a susceptible person
Closed wound	Soft tissue damage beneath the skin, bruises		
Clothes Drag	Emergency position to remove victim in which head, neck are stabilized		
		Dislocation	Displacement of bone from joint
Clotting	The blood thickens at wound site, helps to stop bleeding	DNR	Do Not Resuscitate; Predetermined orders that instruct health care providers to NOT do cardiopulmonary resuscitation
Complete Airway Blockage	Complete blockage of the breathing passages to the lungs		
Concussion	Temporary impairment of the brain function, short term	Dressing	Gauze or pads placed over a wound to absorb fluids
Confidentiality	Protecting the privacy of victims by not disclosing information other than to proper medical authority	EAP	Emergency Action Plan; Predetermined orders of operation and assignments
		Early CPR	Helps to provide oxygen to the vital organs and brain until medical help arrives
Consciousness	A person's ability to know what is happening around them	Elastic Bandage	AKA "ACE Bandage" Temporary covering for wound area with minimum pressure
Consent	Victim consciously grants permission to receive treatment		
Contraction	Pumping of the vessels supplying blood and oxygen	Electrical Burn	Burn cause by electrical appliance, source or lightening
Coronary Arteries	Blood vessels that supply oxygen rich blood to the heart	Embolism	Sudden blockage of an artery by foreign material, air, clot, fat
CPR	Cardio-Pulmonary Resuscitation, combination of compressions and breaths	Emphysema	A condition in which the lungs are damaged and cannot properly transfer oxygen and carbon dioxide
CPR performance	Manual compressions of heart and respiration of lungs to revive or sustain life until medical help arrives		
		EMS	Emergency Medical Service - Professional responders
Cyanosis	Discoloration (somewhat blue or gray) of skin around the eyes, lips; Usually due to hypoxia	Epiglottis	The length of tissue that covers the trachea to keep food and liquids out of the lungs
Defibrillation	Electric current administered to the heart	Epilepsy	Chronic condition characterized by brain seizures that vary in type and duration; Treat or control with various medications
Defibrillator	Mechanical device that delivers an electric shock to the heart		

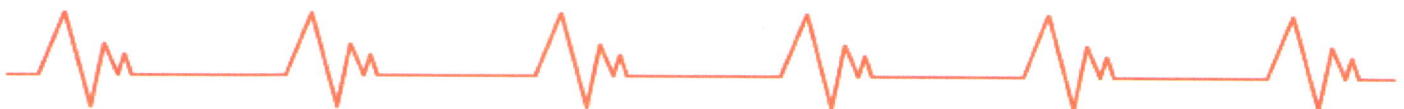

Epipen	Brand name of an Epinephrine Auto Injector; Usually prescribed for patients to use during severe allergic reactions
Exhale	To breathe air out of the lungs
External Bleeding	Visible bleeding
Femoral Arteries	A large artery in each thigh; Main artery to carry blood to the lower body
Finger Sweep	Technique used to remove material or object from airway
FIRST AID	The treatment in which a victim receives temporary medical care
First Responder	Individual trained in emergency care who may be called to provide care
Flow Rate	In oxygen administration, based on respiration assistance placement of mask, varies 1 - 25 LPM
Fracture	Break in a bone
Gloves, Latex, Non powder	Variations of design make sterile non-sterile, powder non-powder, always use in treatment or response
Good Samaritan Laws	Vary state to state; Laws that protect people in emergency care
Head tilt-Chin lift	Used for opening the airway
Hearing Impaired	Persons who are deaf or severely partially deaf
Heart	Fist size organ that pumps blood throughout the body
Heat Exhaustion	A form of shock caused by overheating the body, for example by activity in extremely hot conditions
Heat Stroke	Life threatening condition where the body cannot cool itself and begins to shutdown
Hemorrhagic Stroke	Blood vessels rupture leaking blood into other parts of the brain
Hepatitis	Viral infection of the liver

Herpes	Viral infection that causes eruptions of the skin
Hot Wash	"Immediately after the action" debriefing, see CISD
Hyperglycemia	Usually in diabetes, too much sugar in the blood stream
Hypertension	High blood pressure
Hyperventilation	Breathing faster than normal
Hypoxia	Condition where body does not have adequate oxygen; Also known as Altitude sickness; Can be experienced due to certain medical conditions, mountain climbing, or in extreme exercise
Immobilization	Splint or other method to keep an injured part from moving
Immune	Resistance to disease
Indirect contact transmission	Transmission of a disease by touching a contaminated object
Infant	Birth to 1 year
Informed Consent	Permission given from the victim to treat or provide care
In-line stabilization	Technique used to minimize patients head and neck movement
Internal Bleeding	Bleeding inside the body
Ischemic Stroke	Loss or decrease of blood supply to a part of the brain; See also T I A
Laceration	Cut (or tear) as a result of a sharp object
Lay Responder	Non-licensed person trained in basic medical procedures
LOC	Level of Consciousness - A measurement of a person's ability to respond
LPM	Liters Per Minute - In oxygen administration, a measurement of flow rate
Lungs	Pair of organs in the chest that provides oxygen and remove carbon dioxide
Lyme Disease	A disease caused by bacteria transmitted by ticks

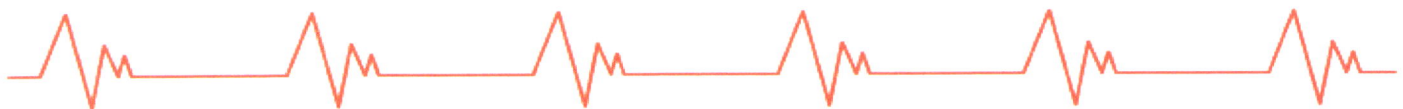

Meningitis	Potentially life threatening inflammation of the covering of the spinal cord or brain caused by infection with bacteria, virus, or fungus
Method of Delivery	In oxygen administration, the choice of delivery method: Nasal cannula, Resuscitation mask, Bag Valve Mask, Non-Rebreather Mask
Mild Hypoxia	In oxygen administration, a lower than normal amount of oxygen in the tissues: SpO2 [oxygen saturation measured by pulse oximeter] of 86 - 90%; Advise to increase oxygen using non-rebreather or bag valve mask, 5 - 10 LPM
Mouth to Mouth	Position of responder to ventilate victim, normal method used
Mouth to Nose	Position of responder to ventilate victim, use closed victim mouth
Mouth to Stoma	Position of responder to ventilate victim; Stoma is usually a plastic fitting located lower front neck, above lower clavicle providing a direct path to the trachea
N95	Temporary air filter for responder; Filters "95%" of air contaminants
Nerve	A specialized tissue that sends impulses to and from the brain
Non-Rebreather Mask	NRB - A device used in medical emergencies to administer oxygen; The patient must be able to breathe unassisted; Allows for delivery of more (higher concentration) of oxygen than a nasal cannula
Nonverbal Communication	Communications without talking, for example use other signs, fingers, or movement

Normal Hypoxia	In oxygen administration, a lower than normal amount of oxygen in the tissues: SpO2 [oxygen saturation measured by pulse oximeter] of 91 - 94%; Advise to administer oxygen by nasal cannula or face mask, 1 - 5 LPM
Normal sinus rhythm	Regular heart beat
Occlusive dressing	Air and water tight dressing used in first aid
Open Airway	A technique to open the patient's airway by placement of one hand on forehead and fingers under upper jaw rotating chin upward
Open Wound	Wound that breaks the skin surface as in torn, cut, or punctured
Oropharyngeal	In artificial respiration, a plastic curved tube inserted in the mouth to prevent the tongue from blocking the airway; AKA oral airway or OPA
OSHA	Occupational Safety and Health Administration
Oximeter	Portable device to rapidly measure percentage of oxygen in the blood; AKA Pulse oximeter
Oxygen	A tasteless, odorless, colorless gas; The life-supporting component of the air
Oxygen saturation	Measure of how much oxygen the blood is carrying v. the amount it should be able to carry
Paramedics	Specialized Emergency Medical Technicians - EMT's - with advanced training
Paraprofessionals	Volunteers or workers who assist Professionals
Partially blocked airway	Incomplete airway obstruction
PCC	Poison Control Center
Placard	Notice, warning, or written directive
Plasma	Fluid part of blood

PPE	Personal Protective Equipment - made to protect the responder from injury or exposures to hazardous contaminants
PPM	Parts Per Million
Pressure Bandage	A thick pad of gauze or other material placed over a wound and attached firmly so that it will exert pressure
Pressure Points	Locations on the body to apply pressure to reduce blood flow, usually where an artery can be compressed against a bone
Pressure Regulator	Valve or device used to allow a hi-pressure source to feed a lo-pressure system; In oxygen administration, the adjustable device at the outflow of the tank
Protocols	Methods
Pulse	Beat felt in arteries with heart contraction
Puncture	Skin pierced by something sharp, a nail, needle, syringe, glass, or knife
Quick Step	Reference to abbreviated version
Radial Pulse	Pulse felt at the wrist
Refusal Of Care	Conscious victim rejects care; Victims have a right to not be treated
Rescue Breathing	Techniques used to provide breathing to a nonbreathing person or pet
Respiration	Process by which the body takes in oxygen and expels carbon dioxide
Respiratory Arrest	Process in which normal breathing has stopped
Respiratory Distress	Process in which breathing is difficult
Respiratory Emergency	A medical emergency in which normal breathing has stopped or jeopardized by allergic reaction or other obstruction of the airway

Resuscitation Mask	Pliable device to cover patient's nose and mouth to provide oxygen
Safety Institute USA	Non-profit organization, mission to help the public with educational emergency preparedness
Seizure	Disorder in the brain's activity
Severe Hypoxia	In oxygen administration, a lower than normal amount of oxygen in the tissues: SpO2 [oxygen saturation measured by pulse oximeter] of <85%; Advise non-rebreather or bag valve mask, 15 - 25 LPM
Shock	A medical emergency in which the organs and tissues of the b`ody are not receiving an adequate flow of blood.
SIDS	Sudden Infant Death Syndrome - The unexplained death of a seemingly healthy baby; AKA "Crib death"
SOP	Standard Operating Procedures; Planning guidelines
SPO2	Peripheral capillary oxygen saturation (SpO2) is an estimation of the oxygen saturation level usually measured with a pulse oximeter device
START	Simple Triage and Rapid Treatment - Used by first responders to quickly classify victims during a mass casualty incident based on the severity of their injury
Sternum	Breastbone; Long flat bone in the middle of the chest
Stethoscope	Instrument used listen to heart and lungs sounds
Supplemental Oxygen	Additional oxygen provided to help resuscitate
Symptoms	Advice from victim on their condition
Systolic	Pressure on heart when contracting

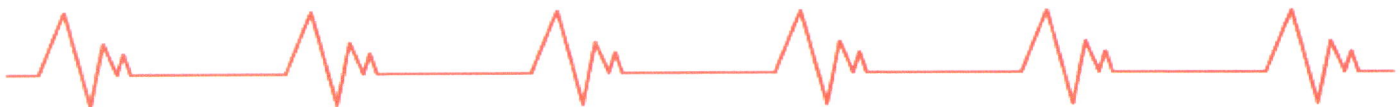

INDEX

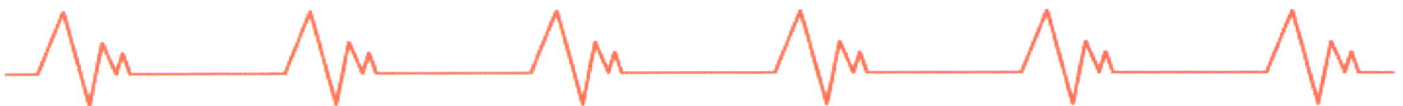

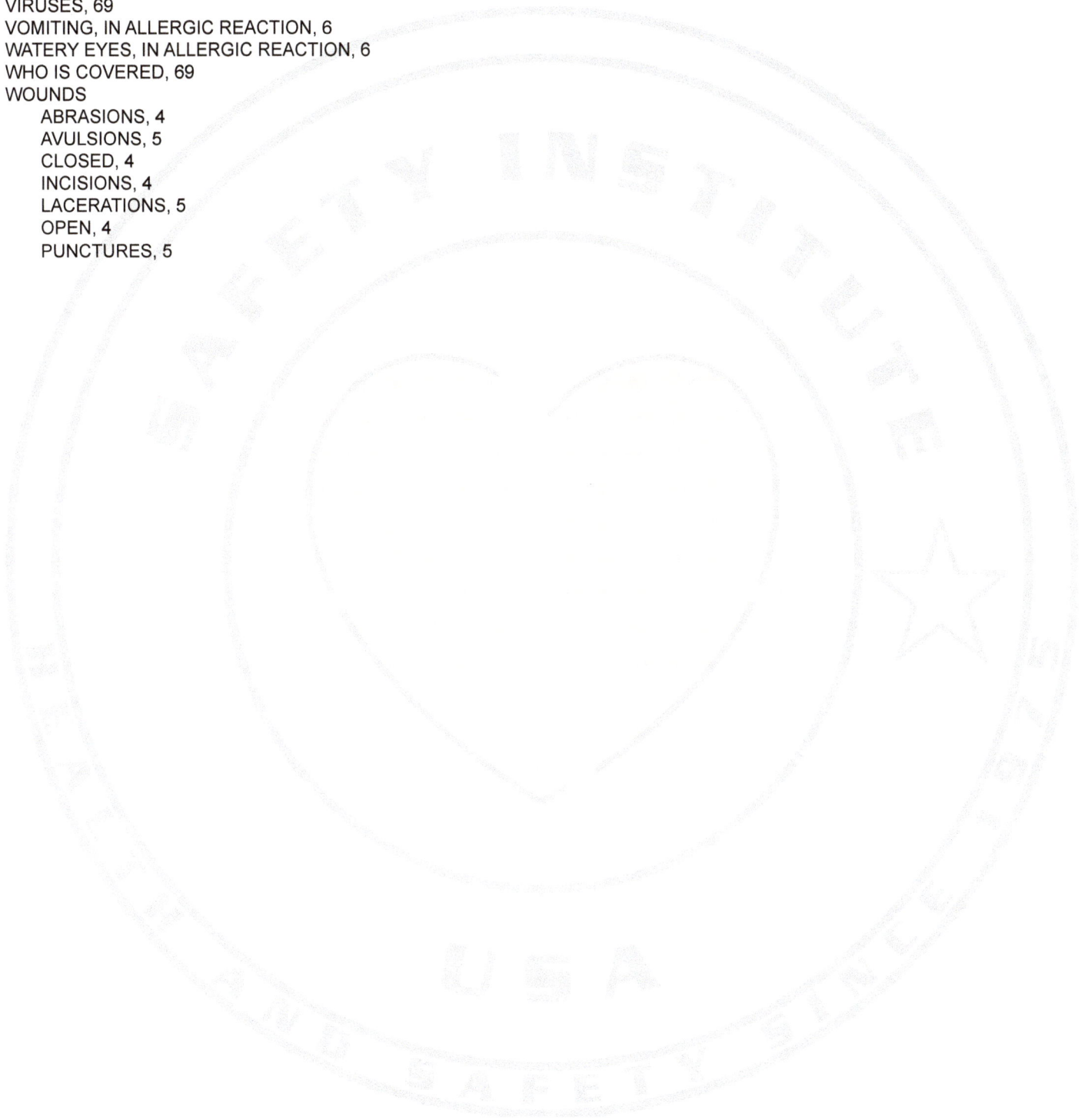

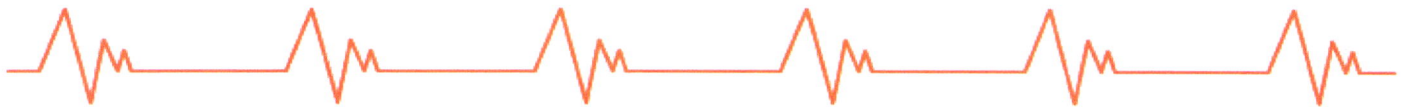

INTENTIONALLY LEFT BLANK

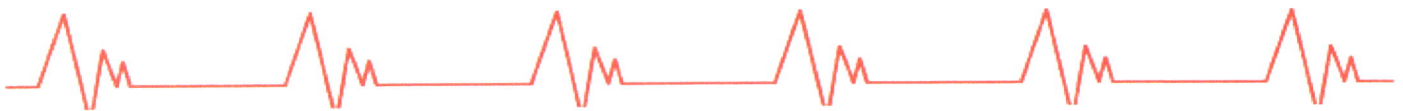

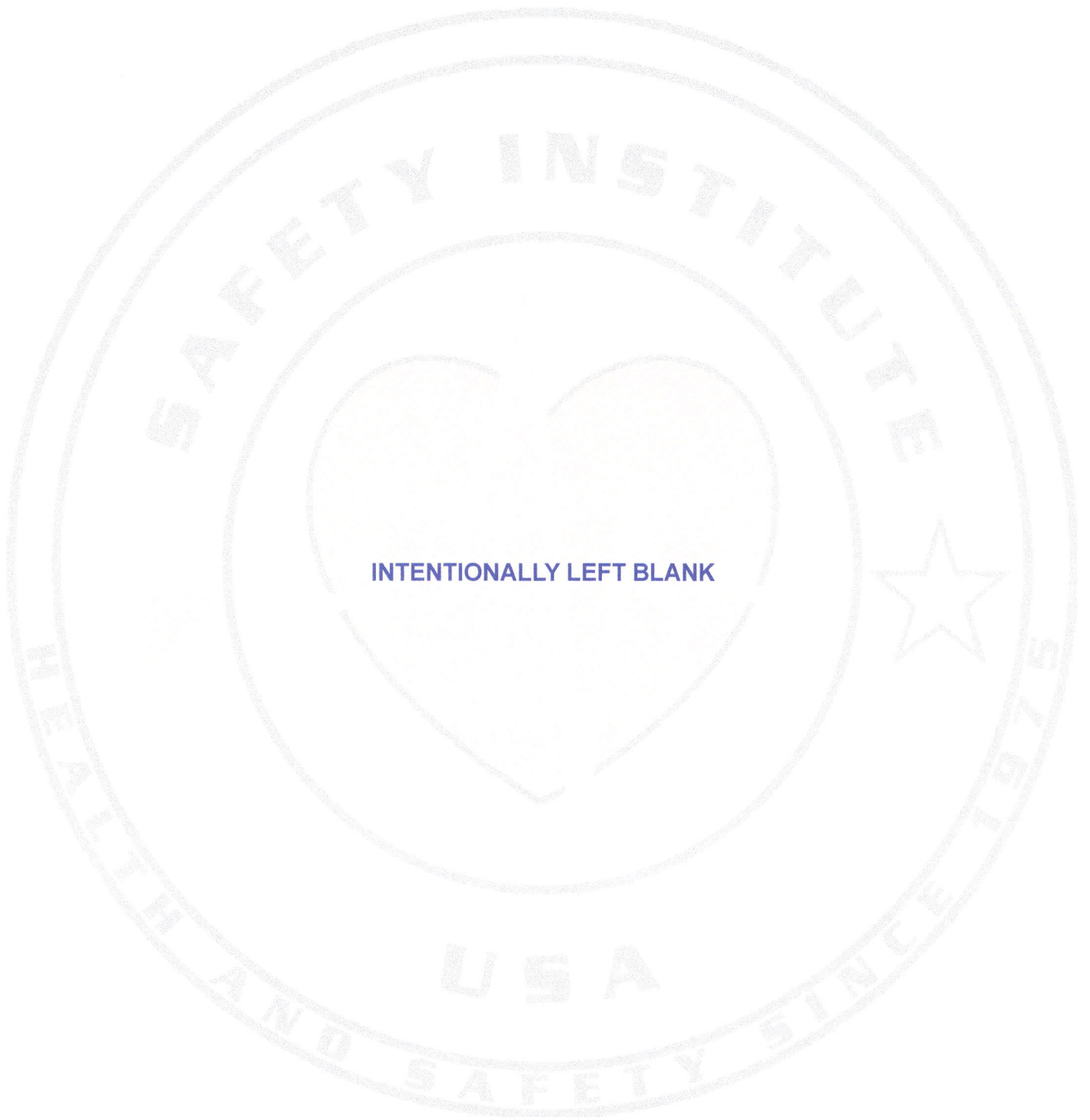

INTENTIONALLY LEFT BLANK

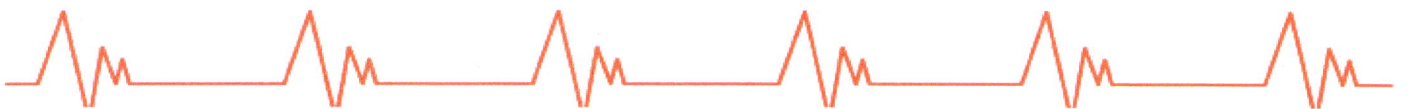

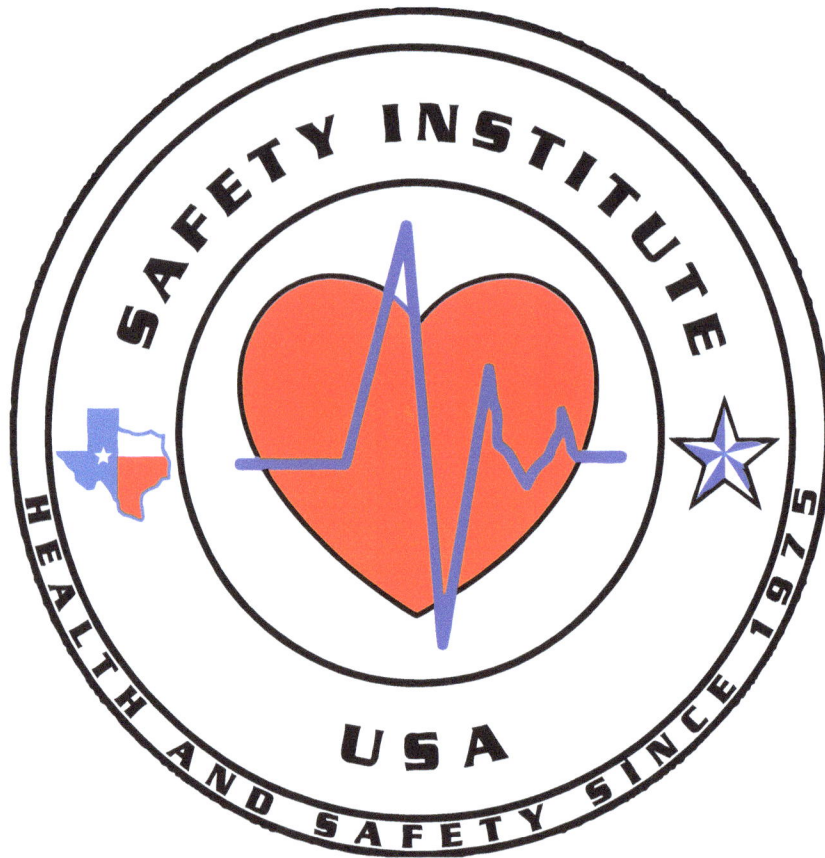

Safety Institute USA, Inc.
P. O. Box 692
Franklin, Texas 77856-0692

Email: classes@safetyinstituteusa.org

www.safetyinstituteusa.org

Combined Manual First Aid, CPR, BBP, Oxygen Adminstration

ISBN: 13-978-0-933316-50-8